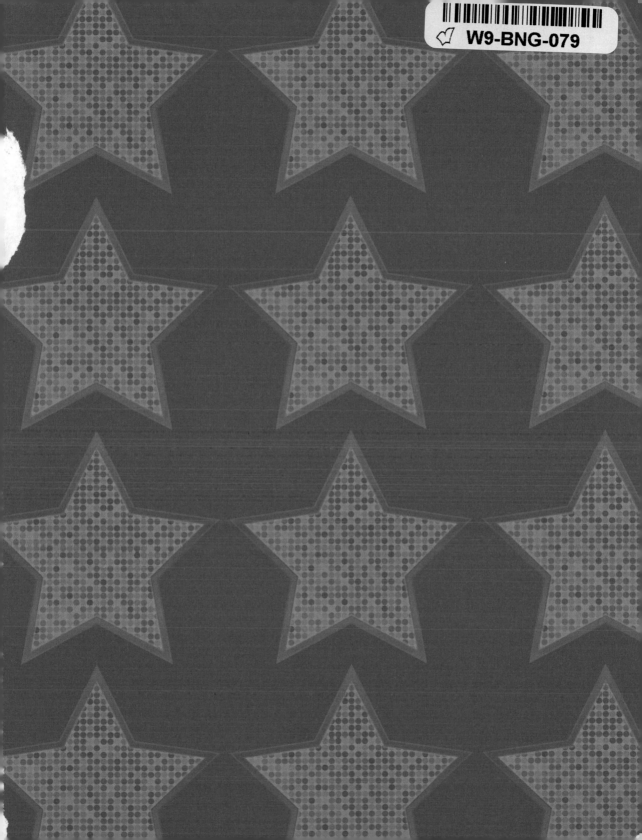

Sugar Savvy Solution

Sugar Savvy Solution

Kick Your Sugar Addiction for Life and Get *Healthy*

by **HIGH VOLTAGE**

founder of **Energy Up!**

Foreword by **KATIE COURIC**

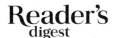

The Reader's Digest Association, Inc.
New York, NY/Montreal

A READER'S DIGEST BOOK
Copyright © 2014 Kathie Dolgin and The Reader's Digest Association, Inc.
All rights reserved. Unauthorized reproduction, in any manner, is prohibited.

Reader's Digest is a registered trademark of The Reader's Digest Association, Inc.

Sugar Savvy Sister portraits by Erin Patrice O'Brien
Wardrobe styling by Elysha Lenkin
Hair and makeup by Prostyle team via Kerry-Lou Brehm
Prop styling for portraits by Linda Keil for Halley Resources
Special thanks to KamaliKulture for providing wardrobe to the Sugar Savvy Sisters

Cover and food photographs by Joshua Scott
Food styling by Emma Feigenbaum for Big Leo
Prop styling for food photographs by Laurie Raab for Apostrophe
Prop styling for cover photograph Angela Campos for Stockland Martel
Food illustrations by Olga Axyutina

Fitness illustrations by Astrid Mueller

Special thanks to the following companies for providing samples to our Sugar Savvy Sisters:
Truvia, Mrs. Dash, Bragg's, Kamut, Whole Foods, Navitas Naturals, and Krups.

Library of Congress Cataloging-in-Publication Data
High Voltage.
  Sugar savvy solution: kick your sugar addiction for life and get healthy / by High Voltage,
aka Kathie Dolgin ; foreword by Katie Couric.
    pages cm
  Includes index.
  ISBN 978-1-62145-135-8 (alk. paper) -- ISBN 978-1-62145-146-4 (epub)
  1. Diet. 2. Physical fitness. 3. Food--Sugar content. 4. Food--Psychological aspects. I. Title.
  RA784.H534 2014
  613.7--dc23
                        2014000512

We are committed to both the quality of our products and the service we provide to our
customers. We value your comments, so please feel free to contact us.

    The Reader's Digest Association, Inc.
    Adult Trade Publishing
    44 South Broadway
    White Plains, NY 10601

For more Reader's Digest products and information, visit our website:
    www.rd.com (in the United States)
    www.readersdigest.ca (in Canada)

Printed in China

3 5 7 9 10 8 6 4 2

NOTE TO OUR READERS
The information in this book should not be substituted for, or used to alter, medical therapy without your
doctor's advice. For a specific health problem, consult your physician for guidance.
    Mention of specific companies, organizations, or authorities in this book does not imply endorsement
by the author or publisher, nor does mention of specific companies, organizations, or authorities imply
that they endorse this book, its author, or the publisher. The brand-name products mentioned in this book
are trademarks or registered trademarks of their respective companies. Internet addresses and telephone
numbers given in this book were accurate at the time it went to press.

Foreword

I was first introduced to Voltage by our mutual friend, Jill Rappaport, shortly after my husband Jay's death, 16 years ago. Jill thought Voltage could help me heal emotionally and physically after the trauma of Jay's illness and death. I'll never forget our first phone conversation.

"Hi, Katie," she trilled, "this is Voltage!"

"Huh? Seriously?" I asked. "Where in the world did you get that name?"

It was from that inauspicious beginning that a beautiful friendship was born. Voltage not only encouraged me to take care of my body AND my soul, but she became one of my most valued and trusted friends. Voltage often says she's a graduate of the University of the Streets, and if that's the case, the wisdom and street smarts she's accumulated through the years definitely make her eligible for a PhD! Through the ups and downs of my personal and professional life, she has always been a great listener and terrific anchor. She has enriched my life immeasurably.

But Voltage is more than a good friend. She is a visionary. Long before David Kessler, long before Mike Bloomberg, long before all the scientists, nutritionists, and public policy makers joined the chorus, Voltage was raising her voice about the addictive powers of sugar and processed foods. She told me that your taste buds are malleable and can be trained to prefer healthy foods over junk. She talked about the importance of hydration and that people often mistake being thirsty for being hungry. She stressed the importance of looking at food as fuel and emphasized that deprivation was not the way to go. "It's not a diet, it's a lifestyle," was one of her mantras. What Voltage was saying 15 years ago (some of which, frankly, seemed a little far-out) is now the conventional wisdom in the medical community. I can't tell you how many times I've interviewed experts who have made pronouncements about diet and exercise and thought, "That's what Voltage has been saying! Where have you people been?"

Through the years, her friendship and perspicacity have blown me away. (I'm always teaching Voltage new words and "perspicacity" is one of my favorites!) But what is really "beyond," as Voltage would say, is her generous spirit. When I met her, she was mostly training well-heeled clients who wanted to look slimmer and trimmer in their designer threads. I witnessed a transformation in Voltage a few years into our relationship. She decided she wanted to work with inner-city girls to boost their self-esteem, educate them about nutrition, and help them feel healthier, happier, and more energized. That's why she developed the Energy Up! program, first at Mother Cabrini High School in the Washington Heights area of New York City and later at five more schools. It's been a transformative experience for so many of the girls. They eat better, and as their weight goes down, their academic performance goes up, along with their self-confidence.

Using her imagination to engage and motivate her charges, she plans trips, introduces new food options, teaches the importance of affirmations and the role positivity can play, and shows them that a big, healthier world is theirs for the taking. I can't tell you how exciting it was to feature the first Energy Up! class on the *Today Show*.

The girls were beaming with pride and a newfound understanding that they could make good choices about living their lives—and that if they did, their lives would improve dramatically. But of course, Voltage doesn't stop there. She even helps their parents and grandparents understand and appreciate the importance of eating well, so she's not only transforming young women, but entire families!

I have met many people through my career, but few as passionate and committed to helping others as Voltage. I really credit her with being one of the founding sisters of the movement to stop childhood and adult obesity. If we could only clone her and put her in every school and home, I'm confident we would see better eating habits and healthier people all across America. Since that is not scientifically possible (at least for now!), we can all learn and emulate Voltage's philosophy of healthy living. Incorporating it into my life has made all the difference in the world! As Voltage would say . . . "Energy up! Whooooooooo!"

—KATIE COURIC, NEW YORK CITY, 2013

Introduction: It's the Sugar, Stupid

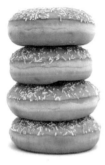

Back in the early 1990s, the United States was in economic shambles. We were coming off a war, stuck in a recession, and everyone was pointing fingers and laying blame. The rallying cry that ultimately pulled us back to the root cause of our woes was simple and effective: "It's the economy, stupid!" We worked together, focused on what was really wrong, and turned ourselves around (at least for a while).

Well, I'm not much for politics (with my "colorful" past, I wouldn't stand a chance at holding office!), but I've been a pioneer in the health and fitness field for more than 30 years and I'm ready to take the lead in solving our nation's current crisis. Right now our country is in a hell of a mess, health-wise. One in three adults is now clinically obese. Worse, nearly 20 percent of our **children** are clinically obese. Diabetes is epidemic, with 25.8 million men and women afflicted with full-blown diabetes and another 79 million folks perched on the edge of the disease with prediabetes. Millions of kids are now succumbing to what once was referred to as "adult-onset diabetes." Despite nearly three decades of low-fat, low-carb, high-protein, gluten-free, vegan, and every other diet that has come and gone and come around again (raise your hand if you've been on more than one), I can tell you there's one simple answer.

It's the sugar, stupid. That's why I created the *Sugar Savvy Solution.* For 50 years our sugar intake has been going up, up, up, and it's killing us—literally. And as you'll learn in Part 1, *it isn't even* *your fault*. Many of the foods you've been told are "heart healthy" and "diet friendly" are in fact **public enemy #1**. They're not only fattening and toxic, but also **addictive**. Yes, addictive, as you'll see in Chapter 1. ***And the food manufacturers know it. It is by design!*** I wrote this book to launch my revolution against this public health travesty—for you and your kids and their kids. It's the SOLUTION to this problem.

Being Sugar Savvy is being hip to the facts about sugar. Being Sugar Savvy is being wide awake and aware of what has been happening to our food supply while we've been asleep at the wheel, blindly tossing what amounts to poison into our shopping carts. Being Sugar Savvy is understanding how sugar affects your body— and, more importantly, your mind—and being able to maintain a healthy balance in your diet. Being Sugar Savvy is finally being free of dieting, obsessing about food, and feeling sick and tired and fat.

TROUBLE WITH THE SWEET STUFF

Nobody likes the word *addict*. It conjures up images of out-of-control, strung-out junkies and falling-down drunks. Only people with *real* problems are addicts, right? Well, not so fast. Nearly everyone I've ever met has at one time or another struggled with overeating. By their own admission, they just couldn't stop eating once they started. Does this sound familiar? Do you open a bag of chips intending to have just a couple and wind up shaking out the crumbs 15 minutes later? Does a spoonful of Ben & Jerry's send you to a happier place when you're sad or stressed out? Do you keep spooning it down past the point of comfort? Do you never feel satisfied? Are you still hunting for more food even after you've eaten a full meal?

Sounds suspiciously like addiction, doesn't it? It's the sugar. That's right. Unbeknownst to most Americans, sugar is not just in the obvious places (like that pint of Chunky Monkey). It is now *everywhere*. It's in your bread (sugar and starch—a double whammy). It's in your "energy" bars. It's in your salad dressings, soups, crackers, and cereals (even the healthy ones). And there's an insidious reason for it— it's addictive.

New science shows that when we take in high amounts of sugar, ***our brain receptors actually change, making it hard to regulate how much we eat.*** Can't eat just one? Yeah. There's a reason for that. Worse, scientists have proven what the marketers (and everyone who has found themselves staring mournfully into the bottom of a once-full box of cookies) have known all along—sugar is just as addictive as nicotine and other drugs. Sugar lights up the same reward receptors and triggers the same cascade of feel-good brain chemicals like serotonin and dopamine as cocaine. And its effect on our mood is cunning, baffling, and powerful. When you're shaky, irritable, and anxious from the subsequent comedown, looking for your next food "fix," you may not even realize it, but you're hooked.

Like all of us, you just want to feel good and have energy for all the activities you do and love. But the foods you're counting on to get you there inevitably make you feel worse . . . not to mention lead to obesity, heart disease, diabetes, wrinkled skin (yes, it's true), and

> For 50 years our sugar intake has been going up, up, up, **and it's killing us**—literally.

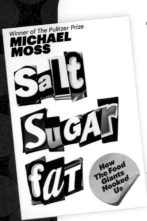

even cancer. That's because they're not engineered to make you feel good. They're engineered to keep you eating! The *New York Times* published an excerpt from the brilliant book *Salt Sugar Fat* by award-winning writer Michael Moss. More than 4 years in the making, the book includes interviews with more than 300 people in or formerly employed by the processed food industry as well as thousands of pages of secret memos, revealing that major food manufacturers invest billions of dollars in a conscious effort to manipulate our food supply (i.e., a half cup of Prego spaghetti sauce now packs more sugar than two Oreo cookies) and get all of us hooked on foods that are convenient and inexpensive . . . and fattening.

A BETTER SOLUTION

Enough! It's time to take control of your life. To take control of your weight. To take control of your health and happiness. To get your energy up in a real, sustainable way. To get **Fit, Fabulous, and Fierce** (my personal motto). Getting Sugar Savvy and resetting your food tastes is the only way. And I'm going to show you how, step-by-step, naming names—both positive and negative—in the supermarket and laying out a guaranteed-for-success program.

I've been in this game a long time. I've been talking about sugar and trigger foods and food addiction for decades—long before it was fashionable and long before *60 Minutes* and CNN and the Mayo Clinic began warning the world about the perils of sugar addiction. How did I know? From painful personal experience!

I was born into a family where most of the women are 50 to

100 pounds overweight. I battled weight issues from my youth into adulthood, when I would eventually become bulimic as well as addicted to alcohol and drugs. After multiple hospital stays and with the help of programs like Alcoholics Anonymous, I shook the booze and the pills and powders, but the food? Ha! That might have been the hardest addiction of all!

> It's time to take control of your life. **Getting Sugar Savvy** is the only way.

I couldn't stop eating chocolate chip cookies—especially cookie dough! I binged on bread, pancake batter, granola (I'd go through a couple boxes at a sitting!), any dough, pizza, Chinese noodles! I would even take to chewing the food and spitting it out!

I needed to find a powerful program. Problem was it was the late 1970s, and there wasn't much of a health industry to turn to! Taking a page from Alcoholics Anonymous, I began to feel that my food cravings were like my previous cravings for drugs and alcohol—an addiction.

But I was fortunate. Thanks to my then-husband, I had the opportunity to visit many top-end spas and state-of-the-art medical centers in search of a way to deal with my issues. I soon started to realize that my highly refined diet, which was stripped of nutrition and loaded with added sugar, excess salt, and enriched white flour, was the root of my weight problem—at the time a minority viewpoint. I began experimenting with eliminating sugar, white flour, and salt from my diet—wiping the slate completely clean for a 100 percent do-over. I figured my regular diet had me sleepwalking in such a stupor for so long, I needed a giant wake-up call!

Then I was asked to become the director at one of the spas where I was a guest. So while I was putting myself through the paces, I had the chance to build my program with 300 people each week who worked at or visited the spa.

I should say, it wasn't always smooth sailing! I spent most of my time banging heads with the registered dietitians in the kitchen who thought I was crazy for trying to remove all the sugar, white flour, and salt from the food! They thought I was wacky when I told them these foods were addictive—that one bite and I'd be binge-eating like a junkie and others would, too. One day I actually caught the staff dietitian pouring salt into the coffee machine! "It cuts the bitterness," was her excuse. I gave her a piece of my mind and she threw me out of the kitchen! But I wasn't to be dissuaded. I believed that I was onto a solution, so I kept reading spiritual guidance books like *The Power of the Spoken Word* and *The Game of Life and How to Play It* by Florence Scovel Shinn to empower myself from within. Around this time I also discovered *Sugar Blues*—the first book to call out the addictive powers of sugar as well as all the potential health damage it can do—which was a huge validation for me. So I pressed forward, pushing the envelope of what big spas of the day were willing to do.

To fortify my confidence and belief in myself during this time, I created daily affirmations and carved out sacred spaces in my apartment where I could reflect and center myself. As I turned away from those binge-trigger foods and into myself, the cravings stopped and the excess weight went away and stayed away. Further testing my food addiction theory, I would occasionally try having just a little taste of certain trigger foods like chocolate chip cookies, only to find that I would immediately feel out of control; the cravings would come roaring back, and I would start binge-eating again. I was convinced!

During those years, I refined my personal wellness journey into a concrete plan called Energy Up! (which is now also a national non-profit organization whose mission is to prevent childhood obesity) and took it to my clients with stunning results. In 1981, I was dubbed "High Voltage" by my friend Jean Kaufman. The nickname was quickly picked up by the media, who

> I've helped thousands of people get their **energy up** and their **weight down.**

thought I was so unbelievably energetic, I must've found the Fountain of Youth—and energy! Through classes, magazine articles, best-selling publications, and TV appearances I've helped thousands of people get their energy up and their weight down. My work has been featured on *Today, Good Morning America, CBS This Morning,* CNN, *Extra, Entertainment Tonight,* the E! network, and more.

Despite the overwhelming success of my approach, my way of thinking continued to clash with that of the medical world until about 10 years ago, when the science started coming out (and it's *still* coming out)—validating what I'd been saying for 30 years.

Around then, I attended a luncheon at Mother Cabrini High School—a magnificent Catholic girls' school located in one of New York City's poorer neighborhoods—for then-mayor Rudy Giuliani. There, I met about 400 inner-city girls, who were being fed the same white bread poison I grew up on, and I could see the future—and it was grim. I could feel all the potential in that room and I knew I had to do something to help those girls live full, healthy lives. That meant my own life was about to change—BIG TIME. With the help of my high-end clients, I brought my plan to the school to change the way children view food, particularly sugar, while trying to motivate them to live healthy lives. I started with kids, because young people are our future. Think you can't get teens to eat right and to give up sugar? Wrong! Teenage girls already tired of battling with weight and depression and bad skin ate up the Sugar Savvy message! All those decades of talking about sugar and trigger foods were coming to fruition! It was working in the most unlikely of populations.

> This plan works because it changes you **from the inside out.**

Indeed, the plan worked well enough to catch the attention of Columbia University scientists. In 2007, pediatric endocrinologist Dr. Ileana Vargas Rodriguez and her colleagues at Columbia University Medical Center found that more than 50 percent of Energy Up! participants at Mother Cabrini High School lost weight, with obese girls losing an average of 13 pounds per school year. Vaulted by that success, in the 6 years that followed, I single-handedly turned three major NYC schools into Sugar Savvy, high-energy institutions of learning.

What was really exciting was how the teachers and parents and school administrators were so blown away by how well the kids were doing that they wanted a program, too! So I started adapting my plan to meet the needs of people of all ages. Now, after a decade of refinement, I've adapted it to be fully accessible to mothers, fathers, families, **everyone** in the form of the 6-week Sugar Savvy program you are holding in your hands. Because if public schools in NYC can change, **anyone** can change! If teenage girls from neglected neighborhoods and areas where fresh, healthy food is scarce can change, anyone can change!

The proof? I asked 17 women of all different ages and with different food issues to try the 6-week Sugar Savvy plan. Their results blew me away! Not only did they lose weight—a combined total of almost 168 pounds!—but they are happier, more confident, and full of energy. You'll hear from our Sugar Savvy Sisters, along with some of my Energy Up! alum, throughout the book.

This plan works because it's not just another diet that you go on for a few weeks. It's not deprivation. It's not a temporary fix. It works because it **changes you from the inside out.** It changes your brain chemistry. It changes your taste buds. It changes the way you think and feel about food and yourself. It changes your life, and it does so for good. The Sugar Savvy program has one very simple motto: **Eat what you want, but the Sugar Savvy solution will change what you want.**

I guarantee it. Turn the page and let's get Sugar Savvy!

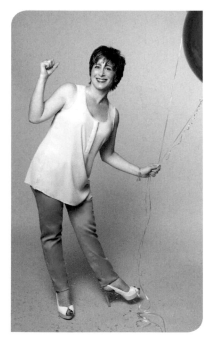

Lisa Brooks, Age 49

Lisa hit her goal weight (125 lbs) after 5 months and is enjoying **"100 percent improvement"** in her rheumatoid arthritis symptoms.

Like many women, Lisa had lived her life on diets. None ever stuck, especially since for Lisa, food was also therapy. "A jelly doughnut always made a bad day better," she says. Because she suffered with hip and back pain from rheumatoid arthritis, however, she couldn't burn off those doughnut calories through exercise, so her weight kept creeping up, making her feel worse. She turned to Sugar Savvy to get control of her eating.

Lost 11.6 lbs and 7¾ inches in 6 weeks!

"I'll be honest. The first week was very overwhelming. The food was so foreign to me and the shopping and cooking and preparing were taking hours. It was a bit of a nightmare," says Lisa. By the second week, though, it clicked. "Now, I spend a couple hours on a Monday chopping veggies and cooking meat and measuring out and pre-wrapping everything into proper serving sizes and I'm good for the week."

> "I don't need Dunkin' Donuts on a bad day anymore. I'm in control. I love it."

As the pounds came off, Lisa's sense of well-being skyrocketed. "My arthritis pain is 100 percent improved. My hands and joints aren't stiff in the morning. My husband and I took the dogs for a 5-mile hike the other day. I never would've been able to walk that far before. I used to have about 12 cups of coffee a day. Now I have two," she says. "I had a terrible day at work the other day and it was a classic 'Jelly doughnut now!' moment. But I had some grapes instead. They were sweet and hit the spot."

Now Sugar Savvy is Lisa's way of life. "I'm not embarrassed to make special orders at a restaurant or to bring my own food to someone's house when they're having a party. If I had a nut allergy, I wouldn't think twice about needing different foods. Why should this be any different? My husband and father are big saboteurs and try to tempt me with pizza and homemade ice cream and French fries. I tell them I don't want it. Why would I jeopardize how great I feel for a French fry?"

Tragically, Lisa's resolve was tested during the program by the sudden death of her 21-year-old daughter. "It was a chaotic, difficult time. But I stayed on track and made healthful food choices without even thinking about it. Yes, I had a sliver of cake, but then I had a salad. It didn't take over. It's been nice to feel so in control even when things are so out of control."

Lisa's favorite affirmation: I am happy! I am healthy! I am kind and generous!

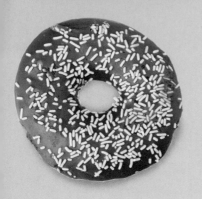
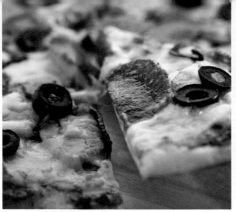
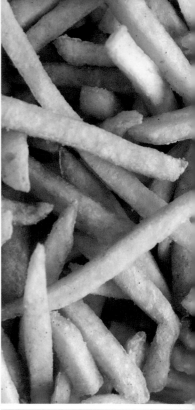
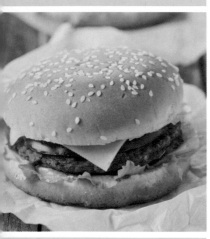
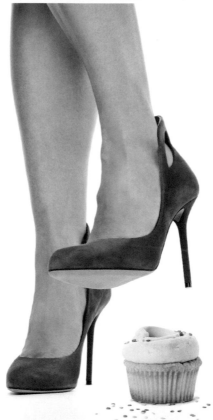
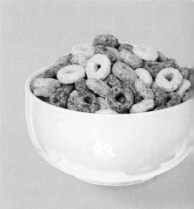
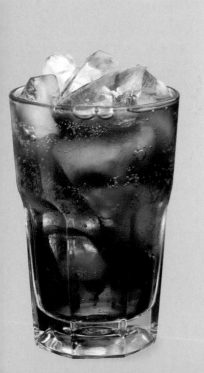
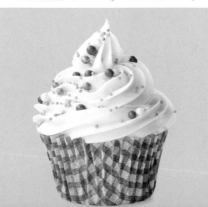
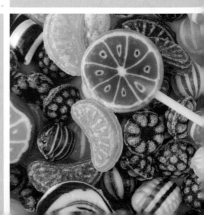

PART 1

HOW SWEET IT ISN'T

I want you to get angry—very angry. I want you to wake up to the fact that food manufacturers spend billions to get you hooked and keep you hooked. The masses may mindlessly follow, but you are not a sheep!

Living your life binge eating and addicted to sugar is like being in an abusive relationship! Women get angry and leave. But then they always go back. "Oh, I'll give him one more chance," they say. "It'll be different. I love him." That's exactly how people talk about the sugary foods they're addicted to. That's your abusive relationship. It's killing you. But you keep going back for more.

ENOUGH. WAKE UP! You will no longer wreck the great potential you have over a damn cookie! Over a slice of bread! You're going to be powerful and in control and fight for the life you deserve—and it *is* a fight.

Sugar Savvy Sister Catherine Schuller put it brilliantly: "We are women waging a revolution against a common enemy in a war against sugar! And we are going to win!"

Damn right. Let's get ready to fight! First we'll lay out the dire food landscape you're facing, help you identify the enemies, and get them out of your life for good!

CHAPTER 1

IT'S TIME FOR A NEW NORMAL!

Out with the old, in with the NEW . . . that's why we created the Sugar Savvy solution for you!

"I used to eat at McDonald's every day. It was just a normal part of my day. I figured it was a normal part of everybody's day."

—CASSANDRA SILVA, 21,
WHO LOST **10.8 POUNDS** IN **6 WEEKS**

"Want fries with that?" Walk into a Subway, McDonald's, Chick-fil-A, diner, deli, or cafeteria for lunch and you're bound to be presented with the same choices: a sandwich, fries (or chips), and a soda. Some variation of this is what millions of Americans consider a normal midday meal. It's so commonplace, most food establishments even bundle them all together and serve them up by number. So when you go through the drive-thru, all you have to do is say, "A number three with a large Coke."

It's normal, right? Sadly, it is. It's so normal, in fact, that we're not just eating it on the go, but it's how we're feeding ourselves at home, and in our schools. Now, with a third of the population clinically obese, obesity is normal, too. Coincidence? Hardly. In fact, once you step back and look at this typical meal that is perfectly acceptable everywhere you go through Sugar Savvy eyes, you'll see that it's this kind of everyday eating that leads you straight down a path to food addiction and obesity.

CAN'T EAT JUST ONE

I'm talking to you not just as a former addict myself, but as someone who has seen the extreme consequences of food addiction firsthand for more than 30 years! I've counseled not just women and young girls, but men and whole families, young and old, who can't make themselves stop eating until the whole bag of chips, the entire liter of soda, and/or the whole carton of ice cream is gone. They beat themselves up. Society makes them feel like failures for being fat. They swear they'll do better next time. And before you know it, they're cracking open a soda and tearing into a bag of M&Ms. They can't stop themselves **because they're addicted**. It's simple BRAIN CHEMISTRY. Is it any wonder that the incidence of type 2 diabetes has doubled over the past 30 years?!

I've been screaming about food addiction from the rooftops for decades! Now, *finally*, I have science on my side. I would like to personally thank Dr. David Kessler, who very thoroughly and elegantly summarized *reams* of this exact science in *The End of Overeating* (though that book was published in 2009 and, sadly, overeating has not ended).

I would also like to thank all the scientific researchers who are finally taking food addiction seriously and are putting it under the microscope for the world to see. Take the latest research out of Scripps Research Institute in Florida, for example. To show just how addictive our standard sugary, fatty chow is, these researchers put their lab rats to the test. They divided them into two groups. They gave one group "all you can eat" access to a "cafeteria diet" of processed meats and starchy sweet foods, while the second group got standard rat chow and limited access to the cafeteria food. Not surprisingly, the "all you can eat" rats on the cafeteria diet got fat—quickly. In fact, they doubled their calorie intake compared to those with limited cafeteria access.

> It's simple brain chemistry. When you eat sugar, you feel a **rush of pleasure**.

That's bad. But it's not the scary part. The really scary part is that *the wiring of the junk food-eating rats' brains changed.* When rats eat sugar, their bodies increase the amount of the amino acid dopamine in their brains, which in turn activates the dopamine receptor D2, which rewards them with a rush of pleasure. Well, when the rats OD'd on sugar, their brain's reward system got used to being overstimulated. So the same amount of food that once triggered that pleasure response no longer did the trick. The rats needed more food to get the same effect—just like with alcohol and drug addiction. Get this: The researchers even tried giving the rats foot shocks when they sought a sugar fix to see if they'd stop eating.

They didn't. They kept right on bingeing despite being physically punished for doing so. That's some scary s***.

Even scarier? Scientists say rats' brain chemistry is similar to ours. When researchers performed the same experiment with people—offering a group of men completely free, 24-hour, unlimited access to vending machines that contained a variety of snacks and entrees like cereals, pastries, chips, French fries, tortilla wraps, and soft drinks, the volunteers ate an average of **4,500** calories a day. That's three times as much as most people need! One person gorged on a shocking 7,000 calories' worth of the stuff. I could eat comfortably for 5 days on that amount of food!

> The more pounds you pile on, the less satisfied you feel and **the more food you want.**

Just when I thought I couldn't be shocked by sugar's toxic consequences anymore, a study crossed my desk about sugar addiction **in the womb!** That's right, mamas, an animal study by Australian researchers found that when pregnant mothers ate a lot of junk food, they actually caused changes in the development of the opioid-signaling pathways in the brains of their unborn babies! These babies were then born with brains less sensitive to opioids, the feel-good chemicals released when you eat sugary and fatty foods. In plain language that means these babies are coming into the world with a higher tolerance for junk food and will need to eat more of it to feel good. Terrifying!

Okay. I am NOT trying to send you on yet another guilt trip—mothers get enough of that already! But this is real. And now that you know, **you can't unknow!** We are breeding a nation of food junkies. Would you ever roll up your kids' sleeves and stick a needle in their veins? Hell, no! Well, you don't want to poison them with an overabundance of added sugar either!

THE PROBLEM WITH SUGAR

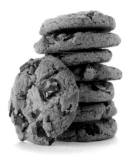

What exactly is all this extra sugar doing to us? The fatter we get, the more immune we are to the pleasure response of sugar and the more sugar we need to get the "high" we're looking for. Like the rats in the study above, people who overeat essentially wear down their dopamine receptors until they're so blunted they need to guzzle a Big Gulp to get any satisfaction from the sugar. When scientists perform brain imaging on obese people, they find that they have lower levels of dopamine receptors than healthy-weight people. The more pounds you pile on, the less satisfied you feel and the more food you want. If this sounds like drug addiction to you, that's because it is.

Sugar also makes you fat. Endocrinology and metabolism research shows that sugary foods interfere with our brain's response to satiety signals, which is a fancy way of saying that under normal circumstances your brain would tell you you're full and you should stop eating, but you can't hear it over the sugar buzz, so you keep stuffing yourself. Regardless of whether or not you're actually hungry, a bite of sugary food primes the dopamine reward system to want more, so you have it, and you still want more. There is no off switch!

Consuming too much sugar also hinders the activity of your fat-burning enzymes, which slows down fat loss and encourages fat storage. Depressing, huh? Yeah, so what do we do? Beat ourselves up for not having "willpower," reach for some sugary food for a lift, and continue the vicious cycle. *The food manufacturers know it. This is by design.*

It gets worse. As my dear friend and Energy Up! advisor Dr. Ileana Vargas Rodriguez, a pediatric endocrinologist at Columbia University, explained to me, "A calorie is NOT a calorie. Your body processes sugar very differently." When you eat sugar, special cells in your pancreas (called beta cells) produce insulin to help shuttle sugar out of your bloodstream and into your cells. Well, if you keep shoveling in sugar, your beta cells get exhausted and stop working so well; that's when you get diabetes.

Emotionally, the consequences of sugar overload are just as high. You get a quick high. Then you crash. Then you crave more sugar for another high, so you consume more. These rapidly changing swings in blood sugar put stress on your adrenal glands (which produce fight-or-flight hormones), which leaves you feeling anxious, moody, and fatigued.

What do most doctors do in response to this? Whip out their prescription pads! They give you drugs for your blood sugar and pills for your moods. This benefits the big pharmaceutical companies who make these medications; it does not benefit you!

IGNORANCE AIN'T BLISS, SWEETIE

This new "normal" is no accident. It's been decades in the making. If you really want an eye-opening (and depressing!) experience, pick up a copy of that book I referred to earlier: Pulitzer Prize–winning author Michael Moss's *Salt, Sugar, Fat: How the Food Giants Hooked Us*. He spent years digging through the deepest, darkest secrets of the food industry, speaking for hours on end with food-engineering scientists, former CEOs, marketers, and so forth on just how much manipulation goes into getting you hooked on processed foods from bite number one!

There's even an industry term for it—the "bliss point." According to Moss's research, a Boston mathematician who used a computer model to measure sugar's relationship to eating behavior coined the term in the 1970s, essentially predicting how much sweet stuff would result in maximum eating! Today, we can find far more calories than we need pretty much everywhere we turn, so companies are taking the "bliss point" to new heights by pouring in sugar, fat, and salt until we "can't eat just one!" Then they supersize it, deep-discount it, and advertise the heck out of it.

More insidiously, even so-called "health organizations" are in on this scheme. I picked up a jar of Prego pasta sauce that proudly proclaimed itself Heart Smart and bore an American Heart Association–approved check mark badge on the label. Then I flipped it over to read the ingredients: It had 10 grams of sugar per serving—more than two Oreo cookies! Sugar was the third ingredient. (To be fair, some of the sugar—less than half—is naturally occurring, from the tomatoes. And the Heart Smart label only takes into account the fat and sodium content of foods. But really, people, in what world is such a sugary sauce heart smart?)

But you have a choice. No one is forcing us to keep eating and drinking CRAP (which is my way of saying **Calories Robbed at Processing!**). You are NOT a victim. You're holding the choice in your hands. For years you've likely eaten the way you have because you didn't know better. But now you do. You are in control of your own destiny. You are holding all the tools you need in your hands to make your future bright.

Honestly, there's never been a better time to get Sugar Savvy. There is a drumbeat for change and it's growing increasingly louder as the studies roll out and more people are seeing how our standard American diet (aptly known as the SAD diet) is killing us and our kids!

Esteemed scientists and doctors are talking and writing about it everywhere. In *The End of Overeating*, Dr. David Kessler got the conversation on the brain chemistry of food addiction started. Dr. Pam Peeke took on the same subject in *The Hunger Fix*. Dr. Robert Lustig outlined the dangers of processed foods in *Fat Chance*. And Dr. Mark Hyman caused a stir with a brilliant piece, "Sugar Babies: The Rise of 'Adult Onset' Diabetes in Children," in which he calls on the government to stop subsidizing junk food, start taxing sugar, and fund community-based initiatives to make good food cost less.

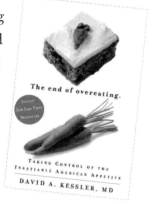

I am 110 percent for that for the future. In the meantime, we need action

(continued on page 12)

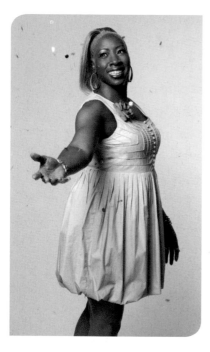

Cheryl Lee, Age 50

After 8 months of eating Sugar Savvy, Cheryl has
lost 30.2 total pounds!

Lost 18.6 lbs and 10½ inches in 6 weeks!

Cheryl Lee, who had just turned 50 and lost her beloved mother to type 2 diabetes, was at a place in her life where she needed a 100 percent life change. And she was 100 percent ready. "I saw what my mom went through over the past 13 years and how diabetes robbed her of her ability to enjoy life. Before she passed she said, 'You see what's happening to me. Take care of yourself.' I need to make a complete lifestyle change—inside and out."

Problem is, Cheryl didn't know how. Fast food and cakes and cookies were dietary staples. She was also in a romantic relationship that left her with precious little self-esteem. She'd heard about High Voltage through her daughter, who had done Energy Up! in her school. "I need help," she said. "I'll be good all day and then binge on Entenmann cakes and Oreo cookies all night. I'm a carb junkie! I use cake to feel good!"

The Sugar Savvy solution replaced the cakes with positive affirmations and real food! Cheryl followed the Sugar Savvy formulas to the letter and repeated

> "Diabetes took my mom. I couldn't let the same thing happen to me."

her positive affirmations faithfully. "It was hard at first. I had to change everything—how I thought about food, how I thought about myself, what I ate, everything! But that was also the most powerful part of the Sugar Savvy experience—changing my mind about what was good for me and being open to trying new things. For instance, I love the tuna salad with strawberries. I would have never thought about putting fruit with tuna but it is delicious. I also love roasted broccoli, sweet potatoes, and Brussels sprouts. These are my new carbs!

"Now I am strong enough to make good choices no matter what everyone else is doing. Like the other night, I was taking my daughter and her grand-mom home from a performance at school and they insisted on going to Pop-eyes! I'm standing in line saying, 'You don't really want this, do you?' They both said, 'Yes, we do!' Well, I didn't want that. So I waited until I got home to eat. The old me would have said, 'Give me a breast with two biscuits,' so I am really proud of myself!"

Cheryl also got up the confidence to break up with the guy she was dating and get into a hot dress that hasn't fit her for 5 years! "Watch out!" she said with a smile. "I'm just getting started. There's no looking back!"

My favorite affirmation: I am happy! I am healthy! I am the best! And I deserve the best!

(continued from page 9)

right now! Immediately. We have all the science and statistics we need! There's no question there's a problem—an enormous, monumental problem. The good news is there's also a solution—the Sugar Savvy solution.

THE POWER OF THE SUGAR SAVVY SOLUTION

How powerful is the Sugar Savvy solution? Using the philosophies in this plan, I have been happily and healthfully living at my current weight (which I'm THRILLED with, by the way!) and binge free since 1979! When I got 46 girls in a New York City school to eat according to the Sugar Savvy model, they collectively lost 70 pounds and got their story published in an academic journal. Then I expanded this program to create the potent 6-week plan you are holding in your hands and recruited 17 women to test-drive it. These women had tried every diet known to man. Many had all but given up! Well, after just 6 weeks, our loud and proud Sugar Savvy Sisters shed a whopping 167.6 pounds and a total of 91 inches! You'll meet some of them and hear their stories throughout the book.

I'm living proof that you can get control of your out-of-control eating and that no matter how bad your food addiction is, you CAN find a way to eat and live that works! The kids in the NYC schools are living proof. The Sugar Savvy Sisters are living proof. Soon *you'll* be living proof! Together we can create a new normal where you're still eating whatever you want, **but you've changed what you want.**

Just ask Madeline De La Cruz, 22, a pre-med student in New York. I met Madeline when she started doing my Energy Up! program her sophomore year of high school. "Like so many teens, my eating was just reckless," she says. "I loved Doritos and soda and sweets. I also weighed about 190 pounds."

Then Madeline went to the doctor, who warned her that she was on the path to diabetes—a disease that had recently taken her grandmother from her. "I knew I had to do something about it. My grandmother lived with us until she passed away. She would get insulin shots and have wounds that would take months to heal. I didn't want that. I didn't want diabetes."

Madeline admits the transition was challenging, but seeing up close and in person just how much sugar she was eating made her change what she wanted. "Voltage took a soda bottle and showed me how much sugar was really in there. I was shocked! No way did I want to be ingesting that amount of sugar," says Madeline, who ultimately lost 55 pounds after getting Sugar Savvy.

> People are finally **waking up** to the pain of food addiction and the horrors of added sugar.

"The program definitely works. If you commit, you'll see results. I lost weight and my energy levels are higher than ever. And it's not just about what you eat, but how you think. Voltage always teaches the power of positive personal affirmations. My personal affirmation has been: 'I am happy. I am healthy. I am a superstar.' I now believe I can do just about anything. This program has been life-changing."

ARE YOU READY FOR CHANGE?

Thanks to all the buzz around new research, people are finally waking up to the pain of food addiction and the horrors of added sugar—obesity, type 2 diabetes, mood swings, and much more. They are waking up to the fact that this addiction does not have to be their destiny. People are ready for change. One after another, our Sugar Savvy Sisters echoed the same wishes and desires for real, tangible change:

- "My brother just passed away from complications of diabetes. I'm prediabetic. I'm unconsciously eating and drinking. It's time to get control and change for good." —PATRICIA NOLAN, 47

- "I have spent thousands of dollars looking for quick solutions to my weight problem and instead have ended up gaining triple the weight I've lost. It's been very frustrating and I feel defeated and hopeless. I want to take control." —ARIS PACHECO, 35

- "I have an all-or-nothing attitude with food, especially sweets. I deny myself and then I binge and my weight and emotions show it! I need to understand how to eat and develop sustainable habits. I want to feel positive about myself and to believe in my own capabilities and start loving myself." —JACKIE GEORGANTZAS, 21

- "I have struggled with weight loss all my life and have finally come to realize that I'm a food addict. I've been on many diets. That's not the answer. I want to live a healthy life. It's time to really change." —NANCY BARTHOLD, 51

- "I always eat when I am tired or stressed. Sweets have always been my comfort foods and sugar control is a constant struggle. I need to make a permanent change." —ARLENE PINEDA, 58

I know change is hard. And I won't lie to you—it takes **time** to prepare your own meals; it takes **willpower** to say no to your best friend's birthday cake or your mom's famous fudge brownies; and it takes **vigilant attention** to root out the sugar hidden in healthy-sounding cereals, breads, and other common foods.

But I think it's even harder to struggle through soul-draining fatigue every day because you can't get off the sugar roller coaster; to feel like every bone and every joint in your body hurts because you're too heavy; or to think you're worthless because you're powerless to stop yourself from finishing the whole box of candy.

Remember that the problem is in your brain chemistry. So, in order to experience lasting change, you need to rewire your brain to change what you want. That's why the Sugar Savvy solution is about so much more than what you eat and drink.

BE A SUGAR SAVVY STAR

Over the decades I have discovered there are five essential points that help people change how they want to eat—to create their own new, healthy normal! These points are the underpinning of my Energy Up! program, where schools hang them on the walls reminding students how to best care for themselves—body, mind, and soul! Consider each of these as points that create a bright, brilliant, high-energy, Fit, Fabulous, and Fierce star—YOU!

Remember, there is a huge difference between "I'm not allowed to have that" and "I don't want that." I want you to be able to say with your heart and soul "I eat whatever I want" because you have permanently changed what you want! The following five points need to become an ingrained, nonnegotiable part of your daily life in order for you to do that.

As you'll see, these five points appear throughout this book and in fact form the very foundation of the 6-week Sugar Savvy plan. It may surprise you to learn that only two of these essential points have anything to do with what you put in your mouth! The others are about how you use your body and, maybe most importantly, what goes on inside your head! They are (in no particular order because they're ALL equally important and you cannot be a **shining star** without **ALL five**):

Get hydrated. Water is the ULTIMATE get-healthy-and-lose-weight weapon! Sodas and juices and sports drinks do not count! You'll be replacing them with eight glasses of water a day.

Eat Sugar Savvy approved. Food is FUEL. The shocking truth is that most malnourished people in this country are obese because they're

(continued on page 17)

Bonnie O'Gallagher, Age 62

Dropped 40 pounds and two medications in 5 months

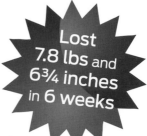

Lost 7.8 lbs and 6¾ inches in 6 weeks

"Voltage is my sister and she has been trying to get me to join her program for 30 years! I wanted nothing to do with it! Meanwhile, my blood pressure was through the roof and my doctor already had me on three different medications! When he suggested another, I thought, 'I can't take another pill. There's got to be a better way.' I just couldn't live with the side effects—back pain and depression—any longer. That's when I called my sister.

"I started working with Voltage at the end of December and rolled into the Sugar Savvy Sisterhood in April. Within 5 months I was down to just one pill and was 40 pounds lighter. Eating the Sugar Savvy way is saving my life. I could hardly get off the couch, my back hurt so much. I have no back pain now. My energy is way up.

"It's amazing. After giving up sugar and salt and cleansing my palate, everything tastes different. I still eat out, but I eat salads and ask for fish without all the sauce. It's very easy. Occasionally, I'll look at cookies or pasta and think 'Oh, that looks good.' But then a second later, I'll think, 'No. I actually don't want that. I don't want foods that don't help me.' It's no effort. It's just how I am. I feel so good. I'm just so happy now!"

(continued from page 15)
wrecking their metabolism with sugar and taking in next to no nutrition. Eating the right Sugar Savvy foods will get your nutrition up and weight down.

Move your body. Run, bike, walk, dance, swim . . . just get moving! The more you do, the more you can do and the faster the pounds will melt off. What's more, regular physical activity triggers the same feel-good brain chemicals as sugar bingeing—and is clearly far better for you!

Announce your affirmations loudly and proudly! An affirmation is a positive statement you repeat to yourself throughout the day. You are what you think! So feed your brain positive thoughts to change what you want.

Be kind and assume an attitude of gratitude and forgiveness. When you do something kind for someone else, you are really doing something kind for yourself. There will always be those who have more stuff than you do. But when you are grateful for what you have, you have all you need so you won't need to eat to feel good. And don't forget, forgiveness is the new "F"-word!

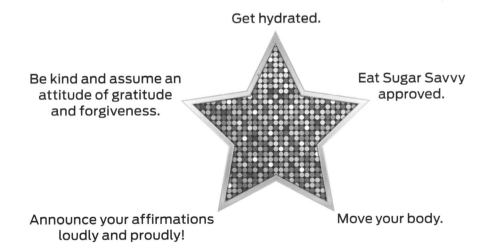

Get hydrated.

Be kind and assume an attitude of gratitude and forgiveness.

Eat Sugar Savvy approved.

Announce your affirmations loudly and proudly!

Move your body.

Some of these points will be easy for you. Others may present more of a challenge. They are all essential for a complete lifestyle change, which the

Sugar Savvy solution will help you jump-start. Sugar Savvy Sister Cheryl Lee, who ultimately lost 30.2 pounds, puts it best:

"If you do it correctly, this is a complete personal transformation on every level. It's changed my whole life! Not just my sugar and eating habits, but everything. It has taught me how to be the best Cheryl I can be on an emotional, spiritual, and physical level. It is never too late to change!" Amen, Cheryl! I couldn't have said it any better myself!

THINK YOUR WAY SUGAR SAVVY WITH AFFIRMATIONS

The Sugar Savvy solution is about changing what you want. That means more than just changing your taste buds—though we're going to do that!—but also changing the way you think, feel, and talk to yourself. We do this with a series of positive statements called affirmations. These empowering phrases, which you repeat to yourself at different times of the day, are a quick and easy way to start transforming your relationship with food. They are also an important part of your 6-week program, so I want you to start practicing your affirmations RIGHT NOW.

Think about it. What are the voices that run through your head? If you're like most women—especially women with a bit of weight they want to lose—your self-talk tape might sound something like this: *"I hate my thighs. I hate my arms. I hate my stomach. I hate dieting. I'm a mess. No one loves me."* If that sounds like a typical day inside your head, you will never be empowered or lose weight because you're defeating yourself before you begin! Your brain is like a computer—it only knows and works with what you feed into it! And if it's all negative, self-defeating thoughts all the time, well, then, guess what you're going to get out of it? Exactly what you put in!

I've got news for you. ***Low self-esteem is a cause of overweight and obesity, not the result.*** "I can't" is a powerful block to weight loss. Negative "I can't" self-talk robs you of your power and makes you feel sad, ashamed, and stressed out. Guess what you're tempted to do when you're sad, ashamed, and stressed out? Go running for the cookie jar, as opposed to the veggie tray, that's what! It is absolutely essential that you be kind to yourself and forgive yourself. What you think and your beliefs about yourself have a powerful and profound effect on your mood and your behavior. Research shows that women who short-circuit their negative self-talk and replace it with positive affirmations are more likely to stick to their weight-loss goals than those who do not.

You can build self-esteem and create a new, positive, powerful running voice in your head with affirmations. They're ways to reinforce your goals, eliminate fear, and turn your dreams into reality. ***Words are power***—if you believe it, you can achieve it!

As you'll see, I start all my affirmations with the words: "I am happy, I am healthy" and then fill in the rest with a similarly upbeat phrase to suit my mood or my challenges for that moment. At first, all this positive self-talk may seem hokey or awkward, but TRY IT. These daily affirmations are ESSENTIAL to combat the negative thoughts that are dragging you down.

Find an affirmation that is most relevant and empowering to you. **Repeat it five times during at least three points during the day:** when you first wake up in the morning; before you go to sleep at night; and at times of stress throughout the day.

You can choose from the following affirmations (my favorites!) or write your own:

* I am happy, I am healthy, I am FIT, FABULOUS, and FIERCE!
* I am happy, I am healthy, I can eat what I want because I've changed what I want!
* I am happy, I am healthy, I am the best and I deserve the best!
* I am happy, I am healthy, I am strong and beautiful!
* I am happy, I am healthy, and nothing can stop me!

You'll also find more affirmations to inspire you on page 123.

CHAPTER 2

YOUR SUGAR SAVVY IQ

All you need to know about sugar (and its evil sidekicks) to be Sugar Savvy!

"I used to love orange soda. But then Voltage showed me exactly how much sugar was in just one bottle—almost 17 teaspoons of sugar! I couldn't believe I was consuming that much sugar in just one drink. That changed how I looked at the food I was eating."

—PRECIOUS CUMMINGS, 19,
ENERGY UP! ALUMNA WHO LOST MORE THAN **50 POUNDS**
AFTER GETTING SUGAR SAVVY

Imagine making a life-sized sculpture of yourself out of sugar cubes and then consuming the entire thing over the next 365 days. That's exactly what many of us are doing each year! Each of us now consumes an average of **156 pounds of added sugar** each year, according to the latest figures from the United States Department of Agriculture (USDA). That is *six and a half times* more than advised by the American Heart Association (which, as you'll learn later, is hardly conservative when it comes to sugar recommendations)!

I'm not talking about natural sugar found in whole foods like fruit. I'm talking the powders and syrups that are being dumped into cereals, baked goods, soups and sauces, and a million other places you wouldn't think to look! That's the stuff that's making us sick and fat. And that's the stuff that you need to find and eliminate from your diet—pronto!

The Sugar Savvy mantra is no more than 24 grams of added sugar in 24 hours! Most Americans are currently consuming about four times that amount—88 grams or 22 teaspoons—every day *without even knowing it* because of all the hidden sugars in the food supply. Even if you never touch another soda as long as you live, you might still be drowning in sugar. A recent study shows that kids aged 2 to 19 actually get *more* sugar from their foods than they do from soda and juice; they are now eating an average of 322 calories in added sugar every single day—enough to add 33⅓

What Does 24 Grams of Sugar Look Like?

On the Sugar Savvy solution, you will have no more than 24 grams of added sugar each day.

24 Grams = 6 sugar cubes

24 Grams = 6 teaspoons of sugar

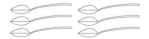

24 Grams = 6 sugar packets

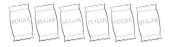

pounds over the course of a year! When you realize that sugar remaps the brain and creates addiction, that's some scary news! ENOUGH! I'm going to help you sniff it out and get rid of it everywhere it hides.

PREPARE TO BE SUGAR SHOCKED!

Let's face it, most of us are crazy busy, we barely read labels, and when we do, we really don't know what the heck we're reading or what it all means. To permanently change what you want, it's vitally important that you devote some time and effort to fully understanding how much sugar is in everything you eat. Right here, you'll learn to be a sugar sleuth. Once you see with your own two eyes the pile of sugar you are eating with every can of soda, candy bar, or cup of sauce, trust me, you will no longer want it!

For starters, here's the math: **1 teaspoon of sugar (1 cube) = 4 grams of sugar.** Remember this key fact. Now, let's get a visual. I want you to go get a bag or box of sugar—make sure it's full; you're gonna need all of it! Now get out a 20-ounce plastic bottle of cola or other soda. Check the label and you'll see that it lists 65 grams of sugar. Next, get out your calculator and do a little math: 65 grams divided by 4 grams per teaspoon = 16¼ teaspoons or cubes! Go ahead and pile or stack away. THAT is what you're dumping into your body every single time you drink a bottle of soda. That's almost **three times** the amount of sugar you should have in a whole day! The New York City health department says drinking one soda a day equals 50 pounds of sugar a year, which can lead to problems like obesity, type 2 diabetes, and heart disease.

Now let's try it with something less obvious. Go ahead and grab a box of one of the popular morning cereals like Smart Start or whatever happens to be in your cabinets right now. Pour yourself a bowl and break out the sugar. With Smart Start,

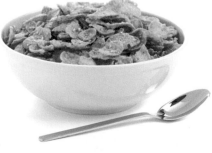

you are eating 14 grams of sugar in every cup. That's 3½ sugar cubes. If that's not shocking enough, consider this: A cup of Froot Loops clocks in at 12 grams. That's correct. ***Some adult "healthy" cereals actually have more sugar per bowl than kids' sugar bomb cereals!***

See what I mean about the power of the visual? If you're trying to lose weight and eat healthy, you wouldn't dream of pouring a bowl of cereal, then dumping three teaspoons of sugar on top. But that's exactly what you're eating every morning if you start your morning "smart." And cereals aren't the only place you'll find sugar lurking. Consider the shockers below. Of course, these are not the only brands that contain lots of added sugar. They're just the ones I was most shocked by. Make sure to check out the labels of the brands you usually eat.

SHOCKER: A quarter cup of commercial BBQ sauce (such as Sweet Baby Ray's BBQ Sauce) contains more sugar than a regular size (250-calorie) Snickers bar.

SHOCKER: A quarter cup of Kraft French Dressing contains as much sugar as a Reese's Peanut Butter Cup.

SHOCKER: Just 4 tablespoons of Smucker's grape jelly contain more sugar than a 2-ounce bag of Skittles.

SHOCKER: Six Dole pineapple rings in heavy syrup contain more sugar than 1 cup of Ben & Jerry's Chunky Monkey ice cream.

SHOCKER: A half cup of Prego Traditional pasta sauce contains more sugar than two Oreo cookies.

Do you still want those foods? Yeah. We don't, either! Here's the thing: Over the past 40 years, food manufacturers have been slowly making our everyday foods sweeter and sweeter. Why? For one, grocery store competition is ruthless! There are more companies fighting for shelf space—and, ultimately, your hard-earned cash—than ever before. The way to make consumers buy is to get 'em hooked. Guess what gets 'em hooked? SUGAR. Remember, they have highly paid scientists whose sole job is to find the "bliss point" that will trip your brain's endorphins and keep you coming back for more.

Another reason our foods are so sweet is convenience. Americans have been increasingly looking for fast meals in a box. As I mentioned previously, much of food's natural flavor is lost in processing, so to make it taste good, they dump in sugar (and salt and fat). Today a full 70 percent of our diet comes from processed foods, and consequently we get 70 percent of our added sugar through these meals and snacks! Finally, and maybe most insidiously, they're getting us all high and fat on sugar *because they can!* The truth is, sugar is America's number one drug!

> Sugar is America's **number one drug.**

This is the part that blows my mind. Added sugar in our diet is now PROVEN to be killing us through heart disease and type 2 diabetes. One recent study that looked at 175 countries for 10 years found that the more sugar there was in the food supply, the higher the rate of diabetes, no matter what the average weight of the population. More stunning: Research presented at an American Heart Association conference reported that *sugary drinks are to blame for 180,000 deaths around the world each year—25,000 right here in the United States.* Yet unlike sodium and fat, federal officials in Washington refuse to set a maximum recommended limit for sugar.

Even worse, manufacturers don't have to tell us how much sugar they've added! Food labels list the *total* amount of sugar grams; this includes the sugars naturally found in foods like tomatoes and berries, *as well as the sugar that's been added*. Nature is very smart and delivers the sugar you need in packages that meter out the doses in a healthy, sustained way. Fructose in fruits and vegetables is fine because the fiber in those foods slows down the stream of sugar into your circulation. Lactose is slowed by

Sleuthing Out Hidden Sugar

Here's how to avoid sugar bombs lurking in the grocery aisle:

1. Always read the ingredients. Remember, they don't have to tell you how much sugar they've added to a product. But they DO have to tell you what's IN the product. ***That's why you MUST read the ingredients list—even for "healthy" or "natural" foods like frozen fruit or flavored yogurt.*** The ingredient list is where you'll be able to see in black and white whether or not there's lots of sugar added. What's KEY here is that you be on the lookout for added sugar by all its names and incarnations because sugar by any other name (and it has MANY) is still poison!

2. Learn all the names for sugar. "Hidden" sugars go by names such as corn syrup, high fructose corn syrup, corn sweetener, fruit juice concentrate or puree, molasses, honey, and maple syrup. You may also see a variety of sugars like raw sugar, beet sugar, brown sugar, cane sugar, and, of course, plain sugar. Ingredients ending in "ose" like dextrose, fructose, glucose, lactose, maltose, and sucrose all mean sugar! Read the whole list, and you might find four or five sources of sugar in one product.

3. Don't fall for so-called healthy sugar! It's funny that when everyone got concerned about high fructose corn syrup, certain food manufacturers started crowing about how their products contained nothing but ***pure sugar*** as if that made it better! It's still sugar, everyone! Same for honey, agave nectar, and other natural sweeteners. Sugar is sugar is sugar is sugar.

4. Beware of fruit juice concentrate and puree. They are especially insidious for two reasons. First, they are made from natural ingredients, so many people think they are healthy, but because the fiber and water of the fruit have been taken out, what you're left with is basically sugar. Plus, they can be in the ingredients list and the label can still proclaim NO SUGAR ADDED because they are part of the product (this occurs in things like fruit spreads or jams). ***Don't buy it!***

5. Note the serving size. That bottle of tea you grab to wash down your lunch likely has two or even more servings in it. The nutritional info is listed "per serving." So sometimes you may need to multiply those figures if you're consuming the whole container.

the protein in milk. It's the added stuff that's the poison. It's the added stuff that has you sick and tired and addicted. It's the added stuff you want OUT.

The easy way to get added sugar out? Make it your goal to eat as close to nature as possible. You'll get all the sugar your body needs to function optimally and be fully, wonderfully energized without the overload that makes you sick and run-down.

COMMON SUGAR BOMBS

You know that soda, cakes, and candy have tons of added sugar. But as you saw in the list of sugar shockers, hidden sugars are lurking **everywhere**. I've been sleuthing out sugar-shocking foods of all kinds for more than a decade—so I've seen it all! One of the very first things I do when I go to a new school is get out my sugar shocker display, which shows common foods with a bag of sugar next to them, vividly showing exactly how much of the white stuff each food contains. Eyes pop and jaws hit the table every time! Here are some of the most common—expected and quite unexpected— places you'll find unwanted added sugar. Find it and be aware of it.

When you look at these lists, remember you're aiming for no more than 24 grams, or 6 sugar cubes, of added sugar per day! We've rounded to the nearest half-cube in the following diagrams. Again, the brands and products listed on the following pages are not the only culprits, just a sampling of some of the ones I found most shocking. Check the labels of the products you usually eat to get a real sugar shocker.

Cereal and Quick Breakfast Foods

It's little wonder so many people complain that their energy "crashes" by 10 a.m.—they're starting the morning with nearly a full day's worth of sugar shooting straight into their veins! They soar for an hour and then plummet like a meteor. Even some so-called "healthy" cereals have tons of added sugars dumped into each box. Consumer Reports recently found that some popular breakfast cereals are at least **40 percent sugar!** You may as well eat a doughnut! Read the labels very carefully or you're looking at 14 to 20 grams of added sugar in your bowl—and that's just for 1 cup, which is less than most people eat. This also goes for hot cereals like oatmeal, cereal bars, and other ready-to-eat breakfast foods.

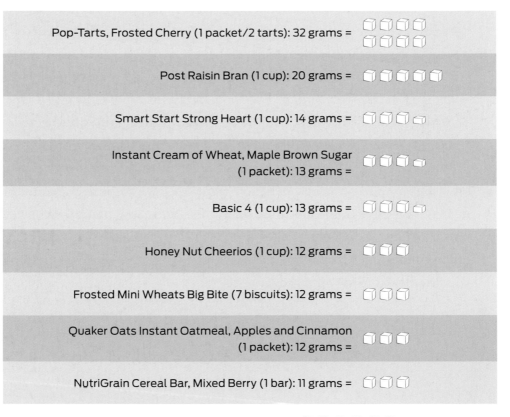

Pop-Tarts, Frosted Cherry (1 packet/2 tarts): 32 grams =

Post Raisin Bran (1 cup): 20 grams =

Smart Start Strong Heart (1 cup): 14 grams =

Instant Cream of Wheat, Maple Brown Sugar (1 packet): 13 grams =

Basic 4 (1 cup): 13 grams =

Honey Nut Cheerios (1 cup): 12 grams =

Frosted Mini Wheats Big Bite (7 biscuits): 12 grams =

Quaker Oats Instant Oatmeal, Apples and Cinnamon (1 packet): 12 grams =

NutriGrain Cereal Bar, Mixed Berry (1 bar): 11 grams =

Your goal for the WHOLE DAY: no more than 24 grams =

Sauces and Condiments

You've heard companies boast that "the secret is in the sauce." Well, I'll tell you the secret—SUGAR! And lots of it! BBQ sauces can pack 12 to 14 grams—3 to 4 teaspoons' worth—in just 2 tablespoons of the sweet, sticky stuff! That's as much as a bowl of chocolate cereal! Also be on the lookout for teriyaki, peanut, and any other commercial sauces. Many are oversweetened. Ditto for condiments. You wouldn't take a tablespoon and start sprinkling sugar all over your hamburgers and sandwiches, but that's exactly what you're doing when you slather on many commercial condiments. You're in luck if you like mustard. Many mustards (honey mustard being the exception) have no added sugar. Many other spreads and sauces can't say that.

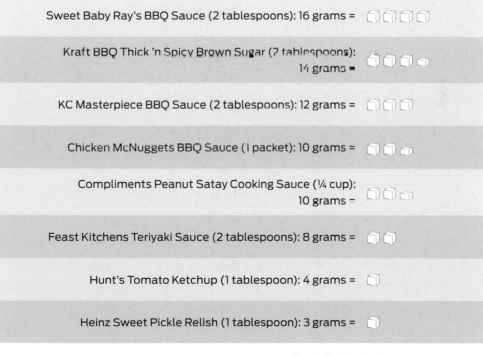

Sweet Baby Ray's BBQ Sauce (2 tablespoons): 16 grams =

Kraft BBQ Thick 'n Spicy Brown Sugar (2 tablespoons): 14 grams =

KC Masterpiece BBQ Sauce (2 tablespoons): 12 grams =

Chicken McNuggets BBQ Sauce (1 packet): 10 grams =

Compliments Peanut Satay Cooking Sauce (¼ cup): 10 grams =

Feast Kitchens Teriyaki Sauce (2 tablespoons): 8 grams =

Hunt's Tomato Ketchup (1 tablespoon): 4 grams =

Heinz Sweet Pickle Relish (1 tablespoon): 3 grams =

Your goal for the WHOLE DAY: no more than 24 grams =

Tomato Soups and Sauces

Sugar cuts the acidity of and adds sweetness to tomato-based soups and sauces. Look for no-sugar-added varieties. You can expect a little sugar from the tomatoes themselves. So don't be surprised if even no-sugar-added varieties have 5 or 6 grams of sugar. Just remember to check those ingredient lists for the added stuff. You'll be surprised what you find. Some brands have double that amount—and that means a lot is added.

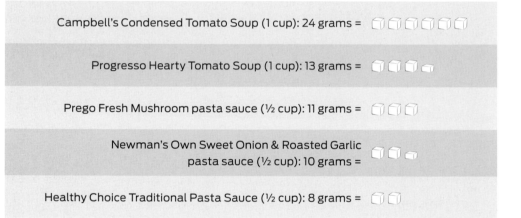

Campbell's Condensed Tomato Soup (1 cup): 24 grams =

Progresso Hearty Tomato Soup (1 cup): 13 grams =

Prego Fresh Mushroom pasta sauce (½ cup): 11 grams =

Newman's Own Sweet Onion & Roasted Garlic pasta sauce (½ cup): 10 grams =

Healthy Choice Traditional Pasta Sauce (½ cup): 8 grams =

Your goal for the WHOLE DAY: no more than 24 grams =

Yogurt

Go plain (I prefer Greek because it has more protein) and add your own fruit. Yogurt contains some natural milk sugars and fruit contains fructose. However, flavored yogurts are full of added sugar, coming in as high as 19 grams (nearly 5 teaspoons!) in just 6 ounces. Be particularly wary of fat-free yogurts, which often have added sugar to ramp up the flavor in lieu of the fat. These seemingly smart choices are anything but Sugar Savvy! You are always better off using plain yogurt and adding your own fruit. The total sugar may still be relatively high, but it is all natural (so your body processes it at a different rate because of the fiber and protein in the foods) and better for you than added sugars.

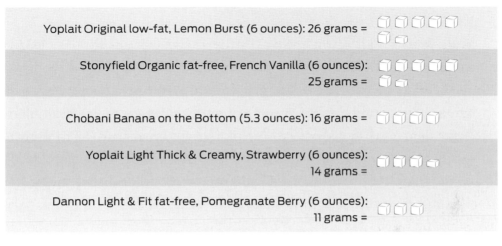

Yoplait Original low-fat, Lemon Burst (6 ounces): 26 grams =

Stonyfield Organic fat-free, French Vanilla (6 ounces): 25 grams =

Chobani Banana on the Bottom (5.3 ounces): 16 grams =

Yoplait Light Thick & Creamy, Strawberry (6 ounces): 14 grams =

Dannon Light & Fit fat-free, Pomegranate Berry (6 ounces): 11 grams =

Your goal for the WHOLE DAY: no more than 24 grams =

Salad Dressings

Watch out especially for light dressings. Nearly all follow the same recipe: Take out the fat, add in the sugar. (Newman's Own Lite Balsamic Vinaigrette has twice as much sugar as the original variety.) Go with simple oil and vinegar blends.

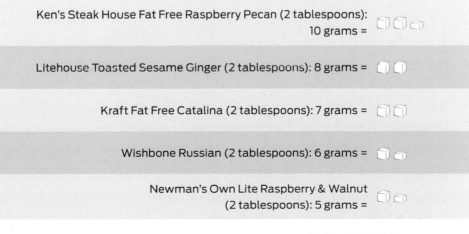

Ken's Steak House Fat Free Raspberry Pecan (2 tablespoons): 10 grams =

Litehouse Toasted Sesame Ginger (2 tablespoons): 8 grams =

Kraft Fat Free Catalina (2 tablespoons): 7 grams =

Wishbone Russian (2 tablespoons): 6 grams =

Newman's Own Lite Raspberry & Walnut (2 tablespoons): 5 grams =

Your goal for the WHOLE DAY: no more than 24 grams =

Fruit Juice

Yeah, yeah, it's all natural, which by the way has absolutely NO LEGAL meaning—I see "natural," I think "run!" Without the fiber of the fruit, you're drinking pure sugar! Many juices are even worse than sugary soft drinks. That cranberry juice you virtuously slug down? It packs more sugar than Yoo-Hoo! Would you drink that for breakfast? (Don't reply if the answer is yes!) By the way, don't be fooled if you see "no sugar added" on the front if you also see "fruit concentrate" or "puree" listed among the ingredients on the back. Fruit concentrate *is* added sugar. Be aware.

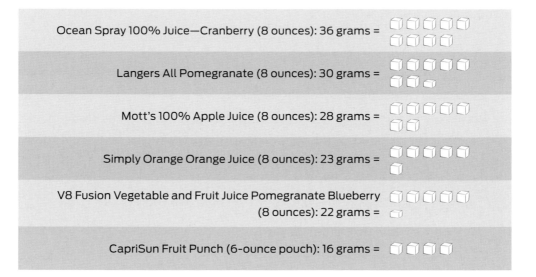

Ocean Spray 100% Juice—Cranberry (8 ounces): 36 grams =

Langers All Pomegranate (8 ounces): 30 grams =

Mott's 100% Apple Juice (8 ounces): 28 grams =

Simply Orange Orange Juice (8 ounces): 23 grams =

V8 Fusion Vegetable and Fruit Juice Pomegranate Blueberry (8 ounces): 22 grams =

CapriSun Fruit Punch (6-ounce pouch): 16 grams =

Your goal for the WHOLE DAY: no more than 24 grams =

Sweetened Teas, Energy Drinks, and Enhanced Waters

These are not virtuous alternatives to soda. Sweetened teas and lemonades can drop a 25-gram sugar load in your system—more than your limit for the whole day!—with every cup you drink. And if you regularly down a bottle at a time, you're drinking quite a bit more than one cup. Here's where you really need to pay attention to your portion sizes—remember that the serving size listed on the label usually doesn't match what you actually drink. Ditto with juice drinks (soft drinks that contain juice), energy drinks, and enhanced waters. All SSBs (sugar sweetened beverages) are the SAME. I still recommend staying away from diet sodas even if they're sugar free because they are typically laden with colorings and chemicals that don't belong in your Fit, Fab, Fierce body!

That being said, hydrating right is a HUGE part of the Sugar Savvy solution. While the best way to do that is with plain water and unsweetened teas, I know that that's tough for some people to get used to. If this describes you, it's okay to use Crystal Light powders or similar sweeteners in your water sparingly. Just remember to read the ingredients and steer clear of anything with lots of added sugars—and stick to your overall daily limit of 24 grams (or 6 sugar cubes) in 24 hours!

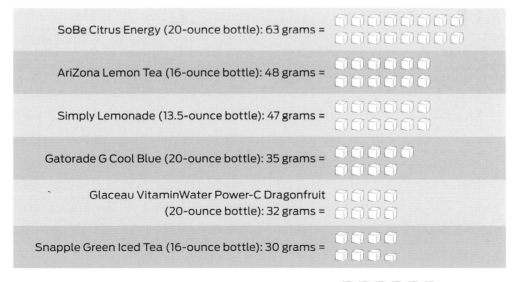

SoBe Citrus Energy (20-ounce bottle): 63 grams =

AriZona Lemon Tea (16-ounce bottle): 48 grams =

Simply Lemonade (13.5-ounce bottle): 47 grams =

Gatorade G Cool Blue (20-ounce bottle): 35 grams =

Glaceau VitaminWater Power-C Dragonfruit (20-ounce bottle): 32 grams =

Snapple Green Iced Tea (16-ounce bottle): 30 grams =

Your goal for the WHOLE DAY: no more than 24 grams =

Energy and Protein Bars

Maybe it won't be a big surprise that so-called "energy bars" are jam-packed with sugar to give you a quick rush. But how about those protein bars that are so popular with the low-carb crowd? Take note: Just because they're high protein does not mean they're low carb—or low sugar. Many are just vitamin-added candy bars packing 15 to 20 grams of sugar (for the record, a Hershey bar has 24 grams of sugar). Many energy and protein bars are also loaded with artificial and unpronounceable ingredients. Ditch 'em and eat real food instead. I see all these otherwise intelligent people swearing by these as healthy snacks! They do not get a pass here, folks. They are bad news!

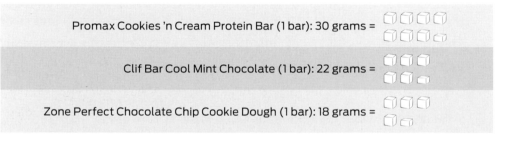

Promax Cookies 'n Cream Protein Bar (1 bar): 30 grams =

Clif Bar Cool Mint Chocolate (1 bar): 22 grams =

Zone Perfect Chocolate Chip Cookie Dough (1 bar): 18 grams =

Your goal for the WHOLE DAY: no more than 24 grams =

Shocked yet? Don't stop now! Once you start looking, you'll have a hard time picking your jaw up off the floor; there's so much sugar in everything we eat! There's even added sugar in bread and bagels—many processed loaves and rolls have about 2 grams of added sugar per slice—and crackers, with some popular multigrain crackers packing 1 teaspoon's worth of added sugar per serving. ***Read the ingredients!*** If it's got added sugar, get it out of your life!

SUGAR'S EVIL SIDEKICKS

Remember the "bliss point" I talked about last chapter and how manufacturers intentionally rig their foods to have just the right amount (read: LOADS) of sugar, salt, and fat to make sure you keep eating and eating and eating? The main focus of the Sugar Savvy plan is sugar, of course. But I've got to at least give mention to sugar's evil sidekicks—excess salt, unhealthy fat, and enriched white flour—which all factor into the notorious "bliss point."

Shake the Salt

Sodium is essential for survival, so it makes sense that our brains are hardwired to want it. In fact, research shows that your appetite for sodium is located in the same part of the brain acted on by addictive drugs like heroin and cocaine (again, little wonder you can't eat just one!). Salt also dulls our taste buds, so we tend to pour on more to get the salty flavor we're learning to crave. I opened the paper the other day to this headline: "Alarm sounded on worldwide salt use." According to stats reported at the annual meeting of the American Heart Association, eating too much salt is to blame for 2.3 million deaths per year in the United States, or 15 percent of all deaths from heart attacks, stroke, and other heart disease.

> Salt, flour, and fat all factor into the notorious **"bliss point."**

The American Heart Association has been warning people for years to limit their daily salt intake to less than 1,500 milligrams, or between ½ teaspoon and ¾ teaspoon—*a very small amount!* You actually only NEED 500 milligrams a day for your body to function properly—that's what I personally aim for. Many people get up to 5,800 milligrams a day—that's 15 **pounds** of salt a year. No wonder we're all walking around puffy

(continued on page 38)

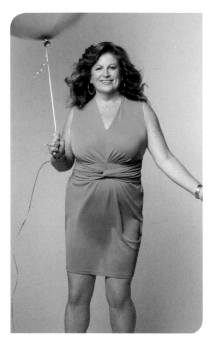

Patricia Nolan, Age 47

"My energy is through the roof!"

Lost 15.8 lbs and 7¾ inches in 6 weeks!

When Patti heard Voltage was recruiting people to test the Sugar Savvy solution, it seemed like a message from the universe. She had first encountered Voltage over a decade ago. "For the first time ever I felt amazing—light, positive, confident—and the weight just melted away. I was a size 6!" she said about her first experience with Sugar Savvy living, beaming.

Then life happened. There was September 11th, which rattled her terribly. Shortly thereafter, her mother was diagnosed with terminal cancer. "I ate cheesecakes like crackers and put back all the weight and then some," she recalls. "As the years passed, things got worse. My brother passed away after a long battle with severe complications of diabetes, including blindness, amputation, and dialysis. I needed two total hip replacements. Hurricane Sandy displaced me from my home. I was on a terrible path of mindless eating and drinking. This program came along at just the right time. I really needed to take control of my life again.

"I stopped having that 'one' glass of wine every night (it was a big glass)

> "I used to say I was 'fat and happy.' But I was really fat, bloated, sad, lonely, and depressed. Now I am truly happy."

and instead started drinking lots and lots of water. I got myself some water bracelets to make tracking my hydration fun! I rediscovered my love of fresh, nutritious real fruits and vegetables. I stepped away from the butter and steak houses. In short, I took back control of the one thing I could—myself and my choices—and started treating my body with a little respect."

Now instead of burgers and fries, Patti is making big, healthy bowls of Soupalicious! "I love it because it's supernutritious and filling. Plus the beets make it HOT PINK! I start my day with a fresh fruit smoothie with chia seeds and almond milk or a scrumptious omelet with fresh veggies. I snack on fresh veggies rather than slimy, greasy popcorn and I feel amazing instead of like a whale. I feel light, uplifted, positive, strong, capable, and empowered," she says.

Now that Patti feels so good about herself, she's also enjoying her friends and family more. "I was so deep in my own self-made sadness that I didn't really appreciate the people who were close to me. I couldn't see how blessed I really was. My friends and family are very supportive of my new healthy path. Everything I need has been right here the whole time! I found the power in my ruby slippers! I'm so happy that I have become Sugar Savvy and will take this with me the rest of my life. I have truly changed the things I like now so the things that used to tempt me have no power at all! Energy Up! Whoo!"

My favorite affirmation: I am happy! I am healthy! I am strong and powerful!

(continued from page 35)

and bloated! Granted, there has been some evidence of late that not everyone is sodium sensitive and therefore not at risk for heart problems due to salt. But no matter who you are, excess salt *does* lead to bloating! Cut salt from your diet and you'll get leaner overnight. How's that for motivation?

The same rules apply when sleuthing for salt as they do for sugar. About one-third of our salt intake occurs naturally in foods. Sodium (salt) is an essential mineral found in celery, potatoes, fish, shellfish, and eggs. Natural is NOT a problem. Only added salt IS a problem! That's why you **must** read the labels. For instance, if you pick up a container of fat-free plain yogurt, you'll see that it contains 150 milligrams of sodium. But if you scan the ingredients, you won't see salt. That means there is no salt added, and that that yogurt is a perfectly healthy part of the Sugar Savvy lifestyle.

Like sugar, salt is found in many very obvious places. It's found in snack foods, for instance, which now account for 25 percent *(one-quarter!)* of the calories we eat in this country. We're not snacking on carrot sticks, folks! We're snacking on crackers, potato chips, popcorn, pretzels, nachos, and assorted other fried, crunchy snacks. And all of them are **salt mines**.

But even if you never touch a potato chip, there's a darn good chance you're still bloating your body with sodium. Processed and ready-to-eat foods are LOADED with the stuff. It's *everywhere*. Canned soups average about 800 milligrams of sodium per serving, with 2 servings or 1,600 milligrams in a can (which, let's face it, is what most people eat in a meal)—insane! Lunchmeat serves up about 500 milligrams a serving. Store-bought breadcrumbs? Five hundred milligrams in 2 tablespoons. Gravies, sauces, cheeses, cold cereals—salt, salt, salt, and more salt!

And don't get me started on fast food! French fries are obviously covered with the stuff, as is all breaded and fried fare. But these junk food establishments even dump salt in the most unexpected places. A 22-ounce McDonald's Strawberry Shake, for instance, packs a nearly identical amount of sodium as their medium French fries! And don't be fooled by price or white tablecloths, either. Frankly, some of the most expensive restaurants in the world pour more salt into their food than McDonald's!

Here are some common salt shockers:

DiGiorno Four Cheese frozen pizza (2 slices): 1,740 milligrams = about ¾ teaspoon

Nissin Cup Noodles with Shrimp (1 container): 1,180 milligrams = almost ½ teaspoon

Kikkoman Soy Sauce (1 tablespoon): 920 milligrams = more than ⅓ teaspoon

Campbell's Harvest Tomato with Basil Soup (1 cup):
790 milligrams = about ⅓ teaspoon

Boar's Head Hickory Smoked Black Forest Turkey Breast–40% Lower Sodium
(4 ounces): 780 milligrams = about ⅓ teaspoon

Heinz Seafood Cocktail Sauce (¼ cup): 690 milligrams = more than ¼ teaspoon

A1 Steak Sauce (2 tablespoons): 560 milligrams = about ¼ teaspoon

Cabot Sharp Light Cheddar cheese (2 ounces): 340 milligrams = more than ⅛ teaspoon

Kraft Balsamic Vinaigrette (2 tablespoons): 310 milligrams = about ⅛ teaspoon

Arnold 100% Wheat Bread (2 slices): 300 milligrams = ⅛ teaspoon

Your goal for the WHOLE DAY: no more than 1500 milligrams = less than ¾ teaspoon

The good news is that once you start eating according to the Sugar Savvy rules, all that excess sodium will disappear from your diet. That said, I know there are many people—and maybe you are one—who have gotten so accustomed to everything being salty, salty, salty that you shake the salt on your food before you even put a bite in your mouth! If that describes you, you're going to have to change your taste buds and the good news is, it's very easy to do.

The Soupalicious Palate Cleanse (page 85) will help a ton. But the love of the supersalty can be a tough taste to kick if you've spent years (or decades) developing it. I'd also recommend arming yourself with some smart salt substitutes. I recommend Mrs. Dash or McCormick's seasonings as well as vinegars and your own favorite herbs and spices.

Fight the Fat

Fat is a complex issue because there are good fats (like the monounsaturated and polyunsaturated fats in avocados and olive oil and fish) and there are bad fats (like the trans fats found in packaged foods and the saturated fat in fatty red meat). From a weight-loss standpoint, what you need to know about fat is this: It leaves your stomach slowly, so it helps you feel full, so you may be less likely to overeat. But your body still needs time to process the signals that you are full, and when fat is combined with sugar and/or salt to create the perfect "bliss point," the urge to overeat often overrides the gradual feeling of fullness. So you end up eating until you suddenly feel uncomfortably stuffed.

All that said, here's a confession: I don't worry too much about fat in my diet. WHAT? you may ask. How can I ***not*** worry about FAT? Because when you follow the other rules of Sugar Savvy eating, it's a nonissue! Think about it. That bacon cheeseburger isn't going to make it into my mouth because of the bun (sugar and salt and flour—more on that in a second), the bacon, and gobs and gobs of processed cheese (salt and salt), and the condiments (more sugar and salt). I haven't even had to think about the fat!

Bad-for-you fats are also mostly found in processed and fast foods. Sausage and bacon and most commercially prepared burgers and meatballs? Gross! A sea of sodium and additives (as well as saturated fats). You're not bound to eat a lot of butter or margarine because you're eating fewer of the breads and muffins and croissants you'd be smearing it all over—AND we're giving you recipes and ideas for far better, healthier Sugar Savvy spreads!

Good fats in natural, Sugar Savvy foods are not a problem. You can eat lean meats, poultry, fish, low-fat dairy, nuts and seeds, avocados, eggs, and healthy oils, like olive and coconut oils. And you should. Cutting all the fat from your diet is a nutritional disaster. You need fat! Your brain needs fat. Your hair and skin and nails need fat. When I see someone who has stripped all the fat from their diet, they look horrible—dull complexion, brittle hair and nails, absolutely no glow. They may be skinnier, but they look sicker.

So eat fat. Just be mindful, as always, of portion sizes. Our eyes have gotten accustomed to seeing portion sizes that are double, sometimes triple, the reasonable amount we're actually supposed to be eating. Stick to lean meats and think of them as side dishes to your veggies. Portion nuts out in a small handful for a snack. Drizzle just a teaspoon or two of extra virgin olive oil on veggie dishes and salads or in the sauté pan.

The Great Flour Freak-Out

Finally, let's take a good, hard look at sugar's most common partner in crime: enriched white flour. I heard an analogy the other day that I want you to commit to memory this instant: Spaghetti is nothing more than sugar on a string. YES! For decades, while people were buying pasta makers and eating bagels as health food, I was banging the drum that enriched white flour is just a dusty version of sugar! It's addictive and fattening and once it enters your system via dumpling, dinner roll, or pastry, it acts just the same as sugar. **Get rid of it.**

People started to get the idea with the whole low-carb craze. But they missed the mark, tossing out the carrots with the carrot cake! Sugar Savvy eaters know better! Flour is at the very heart of food processing. In fact, it may be the beginning of industrial food processing. Centuries ago people used to grind their own grain into highly nutritious, coarse flour. It wasn't "enriched" with vitamins and minerals—*because they were all still there!*

Problem is, because this food was rich in wholesome fats and fresh and nutritious, it also spoiled rather quickly.

Enter the industrial age: We used our newfound machinery to "improve upon nature"! We took giant steamrollers and stripped off the wheat's germ (the part of the grain with all the fiber and nutrients; that's why wheat germ is so good for you!); then took air sifters to further "purify" the product by removing the bran from the wheat (hmmm, bran is good for you, too), and created white refined (sounds so fancy) flour—a nutritional nightmare!

> Enriched white flour is just a **dusty version of sugar.** Get rid of it!

Sure, sure, today food manufacturers "enrich" the flour with sprayed-in vitamins and minerals, which is a nice start, but it doesn't fully replace all the lost phytonutrients that have been stripped out. Sometimes they even stuff some fiber back in there. But, for the most part, white flour is simply a refined carbohydrate. Without the fibrous parts of the grain, which have been stripped away, your body digests it extremely quickly and turns it to blood sugar as quickly as, well, sugar. This sends you on a sugar high—and a subsequent crash—and sets up the addictive eating cycle. So it should not be a surprise to anyone that many companies load up their processed foods with both sugar and flour for a doubly addictive, energy-sapping, waistline-wrecking whammy!

White flour is white flour is white flour whether it comes in a muffin, a pasta spiral, or a ramen noodle. Food manufacturers use flour to boost taste and texture and help make processed food all that much more addictive. As you'll see, many of our most common "trigger foods," such as cookies, cakes, pastries, breads, and other baked goods (like the ones the junk food–eating rats ate in the cafeteria diet studies), are chock-full of flour as well as sugar.

Yes, you need carbohydrates for energy. But according to the Mayo

Clinic, most Americans really only need about 225 grams a day. Some, depending on height and activity level, need even less. For reference, two slices of pizza deliver nearly 70 grams—almost a third of your whole day's allotment. Wanna have a little flour freak-out? Just take a look at how many grams of carbs you get from breads and pastas (and compare these serving sizes to how much you really eat!):

Pretzel rods (2) = 44 grams

Spaghetti (1 cup, cooked) = 40 grams

Macaroni (1 cup, cooked) = 40 grams

Pita, white (6" diameter) = 33 grams

Rye bread (2 slices) = 30 grams

Wheat bread (2 slices) = 24 grams

Sourdough bread (large slice) = 18 grams

French bread (5" piece) = 18 grams

Crackers (about 12) = 18 grams

To be Sugar Savvy, you need to break the addiction by seeking far healthier, more energizing, and *slimming* sources of carbohydrate: WHOLE FOODS, especially vegetables—the most nutritious source of carbs on Earth! Note that even the fruits and veggies that are high in carbs, such as pears, artichokes, and sweet potatoes, are still perfectly Sugar Savvy because they are loaded with vitamins, minerals, and most importantly for your health—fiber. But most are *much* lower in carbs—for instance, a cup of raw broccoli has just 6 grams of carbs; 1 cup of strawberries has 11 grams. Fiber slows digestion, so for one, you're FAR less likely to overeat. (When's the last time you binged on broccoli? Yeah, I thought so.) Also, the sugar and carbohydrates from these foods are released slowly over time, so you enjoy sustained, even energy rather than the crazy ups and downs from pastas and sweets.

(continued on page 45)

Marva Phillips, Age 69

Awoke to the fact that **foods can heal or harm**

Lost 10 lbs and 4¾ inches in 6 weeks

"I have a lot of arthritis pain in my legs and knees that prevents me from exercising the way I want. So I do chair aerobics and water aerobics, which I love because it feels like I'm floating. But I wanted to get healthier and be more active. My eating has been the piece that needed help. Food has always been comfort. I would just eat the breads and the sweets all the time. I was asleep to the fact that those foods were making me unhealthy. Now I'm awake.

"The Sugar Savvy solution is a change. It's a different way of living. It's really been a wake-up call. I still desire foods that I shouldn't eat—foods that aren't good for me. But now I look closely at everything I eat. I turn the food over and read the labels and ingredients and look at the sugar and the sodium and if the numbers aren't right, I think, 'No. That's not for me.'

"It takes a lot longer to shop now. But I've lost 10 pounds, my blood sugar is lower, and I feel better body, mind, and soul. I'm still working to get the hang of the formulas but it's worth the effort. The severity of my pain has lessened and I would tell anyone who is starting this plan to stick with it. You will not be sorry."

(continued from page 43)

IS YOUR FOOD DEAD OR ALIVE?

About 70 percent of the average American's diet comes from processed foods. That is more than in ***any other country in the world!*** Guess what else we have more of than nearly any other country in the world (except Mexico, which just passed us)? Obesity! Coincidence? I don't think so, people! And let's not even begin to talk about all the hazardous chemicals and genetically modified ingredients that are in 80 percent of our processed foods. We haven't even begun to comprehend how terrible they are for us or how many diseases they're responsible for!

> The more living foods you eat, the **more alive** you will feel.

Technically, all calories are units of energy. Your body uses them to fuel your life. Remember that. Food is *fuel* to power you up. When you dump dead, sugar-laden, salty, and flour-filled food into your system, you can expect to be loaded down, belching, and bloated like a blimp. When you eat vibrant, clean, living food for fuel, you can expect to be sleek, sexy, and revving with energy like a sports car! The more living foods you eat, the more alive you will feel. HELLO!

So next time you're at the grocery store, pick up a bag of Doritos. Look closely at the picture on the bag. Does it resemble anything that occurs naturally on this planet? Does it look like it was once even remotely alive? Not a chance. Now stroll down to the deli counter and examine the rows and rows of lunchmeat. More alive than the overly processed corn chip, yes. But alive? Still not so much. Now go to the produce aisle. Brimming with life! Go to the fish and meat counters. See the chicken breasts and fresh fish. Alive! You get the idea. But I want to really drill it home.

Take the following quizzes to brush up on your Sugar Savvy Dead or Alive IQ. Just circle the correct answers for each item.

Are your vegetables DEAD or ALIVE?

1 Raw vegetable salad with rice wine vinegar dressing   D   A

2 Steamed asparagus with lemon and tarragon   D   A

3 Frozen creamed spinach   D   A

4 Canned baby peas and carrots   D   A

5 Baked potato   D   A

6 Grated red cabbage and carrots   D   A

7 Frozen Tater Tots   D   A

8 Deli coleslaw   D   A

9 Frozen (unsauced) steam-in-the-bag green beans   D   A

Answers

ALIVE: 1, 2, 5, 6, 9. These are examples of how you should take your veggies: straight, in salads, steamed, freshly grated, or baked, with all the nutrients intact. Frozen veggies are perfectly fine, so long as they are not processed (like Tater Tots) or smothered in sauces.

DEATH TOLL: 3, 4, 7, 8. Being processed, breaded, or doused in cream sauce, locked up and sealed in a can, or drenched in salt and mayo kills your poor veggies. Let them live!

Are your fruits DEAD or ALIVE?

1 Canned peaches in light syrup   D   A

2 McIntosh apples   D   A

3 Frozen blueberries   D   A

4 Jar of applesauce   D   A

5 Banana, just peeled   D   A

6 Slice of watermelon   D   A

7 Cherry pie   D   A

8 Homemade fruit puree (no sugar added)   D   A

Answers

ALIVE: 2, 3, 5, 6, 8. You want your fruit fresh and juicy. Once you get your taste buds hooked on the real thing, there's no going back to the alternative. In the case of frozen fruits, remember to read the labels. Fresh is best. But frozen is perfectly okay so long as there is ZERO sugar added.

DEATH TOLL: 1, 4, 7. Canned and jarred fruits are generally overwhelmed with sugary syrups, additives, and preservatives. If you find a cherry pie—especially a store-bought one—that hasn't been drowned in sugar, if not syrup and starch, let me know and I'll eat it myself!

Are your meats and fish DEAD or ALIVE?

1	Organic beefsteak	D	A
2	Frozen Salisbury steak dinner	D	A
3	Sashimi	D	A
4	Frozen breaded fish fillets	D	A
5	Deli turkey roll	D	A
6	Smoked salmon	D	A
7	Frozen breakfast sausages	D	A
8	Fresh trout, broiled and splashed with lemon	D	A

Answers

ALIVE: 1, 3, 8. Your meats, poultries, and fish should be FRESH—ALWAYS.

DEATH TOLL: 2, 4, 5, 6, 7. Watch out for all the "fatal" salt traps in these foods. Frozen dinners, breading, and the smoking and processing required to make cold cuts all kill the vitality in the food before you eat it.

Are your snacks DEAD or ALIVE?

1	Glazed doughnut	D	A
2	Fat-free Velveeta	D	A
3	Three Musketeers chocolate bar	D	A
4	Bag of chips	D	A
5	Slice of mushroom pizza	D	A
6	Fresh strawberries	D	A
7	Crackers and cheese snack pack	D	A
8	Crudités with homemade salsa	D	A

Answers

ALIVE: 6, 8. This should've been a gimme, folks. If it doesn't look alive—IT'S DEAD. The mushrooms are the only thing remotely alive in the rest of the selections, and even they are likely cooked within an inch of their lives!

DEATH TOLL: 1, 2, 3, 4, 5, 7. Lots of sugar, salt, fat, and flour smothering any semblance of real Sugar Savvy foods here! Fortunately, once you get a taste for the real thing, you won't want any of these DOA foods any longer!

CHAPTER 3

PULL THE TRIGGERS

*Time to kick your trigger foods to the curb—
and to always be prepared for when "life happens"!*

"I'm very disciplined about working out. I do triathlons, so I run and swim and ride my bike. But you would never know it to see me. I don't look like the athlete I am. That's because I'm a food addict. I can easily erase a full day of activity by sitting down in the evening with a carton of ice cream. I sit there beating myself up, because it's so frustrating to undo all my hard work because I can't stop eating."

—NANCY BARTHOLD, 51,
WHO LOST **11.2 POUNDS** IN **6 WEEKS**

Sound familiar? I bet it does. Time to look in the mirror and be painfully honest with yourself: Are there any foods you simply cannot eat just one (or two or three) of? If you're holding this book in your hands, I know the answer is YES. Each of us has foods that we simply cannot eat in reasonable amounts. When we have one bite, we want more, and the urge to overeat begins.

Take, for instance, one of my Energy Up! girls, a young lady named Precious. When I first met Precious, she was carrying about 50 unwanted pounds and, though she was just 15, she could barely walk up the hill to her school. In fact, by her own admission, she **couldn't** make it up the hill to her school without stopping multiple times. Precious didn't know it then, but she was hopelessly addicted to sugar.

"I would buy 15 packs of Twizzlers a day. And I drank a *lot* of soda—about three bottles a day. I loved potato chips and fried chicken. I was steadily putting on weight, but I didn't even realize it," she recalls. "I just know I was tired all the time, so I kept eating the candy and drinking the soda for a lift." That "lift" was an anchor in disguise! Precious not only ended up drained of all her energy, but her weight climbed to 180 as her confidence and self-worth sank to all-time lows. "My cousins would call me fat and it would really get me down. I just didn't feel very good about myself."

We are hardwired to **want trigger foods.** And food manufacturers know it.

Or how about Cheryl Lee, 50, who knew she had to change her ways after her mother's death from diabetes complications yet **still** could not resist the pull of SUGAR. "I'm a binge eater. I'll be so good and careful and watch what I eat and then at night I'll start in with the Entenmann's cakes and the Oreos and I'll keep eating until they're gone."

Or Perri Blumberg, 24, who as a former psych major KNOWS all too well about sugar's addictive powers yet **still** can't kick the habit. "One mere bite of a delectably delicate, perfectly flavored sea salt and vinegar chip for me means the whole jumbo bag. Just a single bite of a devilishly alluring cookie beckons me to keep eating until I have devoured the whole box. My brain simply does not understand the concept of 'just one taste.'"

CAN'T FIND THE OFF SWITCH!

I'm going to bet that like me, the women above, and every client I've ever seen, you have foods that send you into a state of out-of-control eating. One bite and you're funked, as we say. You mean to have just one spoonful of Nutella and suddenly you're scraping the bottom of the jar. You intend to have just a few French fries, a small sliver of cheesecake, or a tiny handful of M&Ms only to end up, once again, eating them all and feeling like a failure. There is simply no off switch!

It is not your fault. These are called "trigger foods" for a reason! We all have them. We are hardwired to want them. And food manufacturers know it. Here's how it works: You see the plate of cookies (or smell them, or read about them) and your brain, trained like Pavlov's dog to crave sugar, simply won't leave you alone till you take *just one cookie*. It's what Dr. David Kessler refers to as "cue-induced wanting." Your brain has learned the association between sugar and pleasure. You don't even need to taste the food to be overwhelmed by desire. The mere sight of a slice of chocolate cake—even if it's just a picture on a billboard—trips your brain's sensors and cues the cravings. This is true for everyone, but in some of us, unfortunately, the effect is more powerful and the urges are stronger. Again, it's the dopamine talking. Trigger foods—just like martinis and drugs— light up the dopamine pathway in your brain, which is a neural highway straight toward PLEASUREVILLE. In lab studies, rats given access to Oreos or cocaine actually preferred the cookies to cocaine. Think about it!

You take a bite. Just one bite. And whoosh, you get a rush of dopamine. Problem is, you've just opened the floodgates. Your brain, high on dope—I

Identify Your Own Trigger Foods

Now that you have an idea of what types of foods can trigger your addiction, take a moment to think about the specific foods that you just can't stop eating once you start. Doritos? Chocolate chip cookies? Any kind of pasta? Write them down:

_____

_____

_____

_____

_____

Next, start reprogramming your mind. Tell yourself that you don't want these foods anymore because they are nasty! My trigger foods included cookies, cakes, and all sorts of baked goods. But I trained myself to think of buttery and cinnamon-y smells as dog poo. You don't have to go to that extreme, but find your own imagery to remind yourself that your trigger foods aren't good for you.

mean DOP-A-MINE—wants more—**now**. Meanwhile, in your bloodstream, your nervous system delivers a shot of insulin to reel in your blood sugar (which then drops as quickly as it rose). The more times you repeat this cycle, the more entrenched those pleasure pathways become, the easier it is to trip them, and the more food it takes to satisfy them.

As we talked about in Chapter 1, these episodes of out-of-control eating never happen with spinach or apples, but only with sugary, salty, fatty, flour-filled foods. Just as cocaine and marijuana start out as plants, but are processed to enhance the drug-like effects, so has our modern food supply been processed to have greater amounts of sugar, salt, enriched white flour, and unhealthy fat. The combined punch of these additives not only impairs your brain's ability to regulate appetite and cravings—so you don't even register that you've eaten a whole tray full of food until you're stuffed to the gills!—but the sugar boosts your levels of ghrelin, the hormone responsible for increasing appetite. Is it any wonder that "you can't eat just one"??

THE TRIGGER FOOD TRAP QUIZ

Just as some people can drink just a little alcohol, there are people who are less susceptible to the addictive pulls of food. Some people can have bags of potato chips in the house till they go stale from neglect, but can't leave ice cream in the freezer without it disappearing in a single sitting. Trigger foods tend to be very personal. You probably have some idea of what foods may be problematic for you, but this quiz, based on my personal experience with the Energy Up! students, their families, and other clients over the years, will help you zero in on them. Answer yes or no.

1 If you reach for one cookie or chip, is the bag empty before you know it?   Y   N

2 Can you easily skip dessert, but empty the bread basket— and the pasta platter?   Y   N

3 Can you control your food intake during meals, but lose it when you start to snack, especially on chips and crackers?   Y   N

4 When you want to lose weight, is it easier to skip meals altogether rather than just eat smaller ones?   Y   N

5 Are you tired all the time? Are there things you'd love to do, but you just don't have the energy?   Y   N

6 Once you've had "just a taste" of bread, bagels, muffins, crackers, pasta, and rice, do you keep going back for second (or third) helpings?   Y   N

7 Do you spend the day on a roller coaster of snacking highs and lows, hitting the doughnuts in the morning, the vending machine chips or candy in the afternoon, and the ice cream at night?   Y   N

8 Do you eat healthy when around other people, but lose it when you're alone?   Y   N

If you answered *Yes* to two or more odd-numbered questions, your food addiction likely lies with sweets and/or salty snacks—those foods like cookies, chips, and cakes—that have been carefully engineered to keep you eating and eating and eating. Once you've reached your goal weight, you can likely add back some grain-based foods like whole grain bread, but you'll need to find snacks and desserts that don't set you off. Even then, though, I suggest that you avoid keeping them in your house; just enjoy a few occasionally when you go out.

If you answered *Yes* to two or more even-numbered questions, you are highly susceptible to the addictive powers of white flour (which, remember, acts a whole lot like sugar in your system) wherever it is found! Like me (and more than a few members of our Sugar Savvy test team), you need to kick all refined foods to the curb, probably permanently. Since desserts and snacks are not always a problem, you may be able to cautiously add back certain "treats" that are not triggers for you. But it may take a little trial and error and I do not recommend it until you have been at your goal weight for a few months.

If you answered *Yes* to two or more odd- and even-numbered questions (i.e., four total questions), you, like me, are highly susceptible to food addiction, period! That means you're in danger of overeating pretty much all "bliss point" types of foods. But don't despair! Your life is going to completely change once you start living Sugar Savvy!

THE ALL-NATURAL HIGH

No matter where you fall on the food addiction scale—whether one bite of darn near anything sends you into a kitchen-clearing food bender or you have just a few choice triggers that trip your reward center into overdrive—you need to toss out the old, energy-sapping, disease-causing, sugary, fatty, low-nutrition junk and replace it with a new natural high in the form of Sugar Savvy foods!

Any foods that trigger an eating binge are not your friend. They are not something you want in your life. The Sugar Savvy solution will help you get them out—permanently! The Sugar Savvy solution isn't about willpower. Willpower always gives out eventually. The Sugar Savvy solution is not about saying, "I can't have that." Because when you say, "I can't have it," you'll eventually give in and have it all and then some.

> The Sugar Savvy solution is about saying, **"I don't want that!"**

The Sugar Savvy solution is about saying, "I don't want that!" I don't want to hate how I feel and hate how I look because of some cheap boxed cake. I don't want to have zero energy and be sick all the time because of a bunch of crappy cookies. It's changing the way you look at food. Changing your relationship with food. Being able to say, "I don't want that," and walk away. When you're Sugar Savvy, that's exactly what you'll do. You'll eat what you want, but you'll change what you want.

The girls, women, and families I've worked with—even the most hard-core addicts—are shocked at how quickly their taste buds can change and make even lifelong cravings go away! You'll not only find a newfound freedom from food obsession, but you will emerge a more energetic, lighter, leaner you, or, as we say, you'll be Fit, Fab, and Fierce!

After I showed her how much sugar was in the orange sodas she was downing (nearly 17 teaspoons per bottle, if you've forgotten!), Precious recalls, "I was stunned. I couldn't believe I was putting that much sugar into my body—plus the Twizzlers! I knew I didn't want that anymore. I told my mom I wanted to start eating healthy. So instead of fried chicken, we had baked chicken and we'd eat more peppers instead of all the rice. I stopped the soda and started drinking nothing but water. No more chips, candy, and junk food. I didn't want it after I saw what was really in it."

Precious saw improvements IMMEDIATELY. "My energy went up right away. I was sleeping better and feeling better. I started losing weight and eventually lost about 50 pounds. That hill on the way to school? I have no problem walking up and down it anymore. I have tons of confidence and feel beautiful the way I am."

Once you make that connection, there's no turning back. One after another, our Sugar Savvy Sisters found themselves marching away from their unhealthy food habits and addictions and into the light—and got lighter in the process! "I was so tired all the time—just no energy," recalls Yoselis Balbi, 38, one of the Sugar Savvy Sisters who tested this program. "It never occurred to me that it was my diet! I lived on carbs and bread—and it was killing me! I could barely walk down the block without resting. I never imagined sugar could make you feel so bad! Or that getting rid of it could make you feel so great!"

TRIGGER FEELINGS: STOP WHAT SETS YOU OFF!

Okay. Time to dig a little deeper! The out-of-control binge that follows a bite of trigger foods is about the effect of the food, not about *you* personally. But let's face it: Very often there is a **trigger feeling** that sends you on the hunt for those chips, cookies, and other trigger foods. STOP! When you're out there hunting for a sugar high, it's usually not because you're hungry. It's because you're looking to self-medicate! But here's the thing: Your emotions may be the reason you go hunting for ice cream, but they're *not* the reason you can not stop eating.

So many Sugar Savvy Sisters would say, "Voltage, but I had a terrible review at work so of course I opened a bag of chips when I got home!" Or "My boyfriend and I had a fight. I needed the ice cream!" To that I say, YES, you have emotions that make you want to eat. Go ahead and eat. But eat the *right* foods, *not* the ones that trigger a binge. You need to stop connecting your emotional eating with immediately reaching for CRAP (Calories Robbed at Processing). As part of this program you will have Sugar Savvy snacks that you should carry with you **at all times**, so you are prepared when life happens and you want to eat! Because you can still eat. You're just going to change **_what_** you're eating. For instance, I don't leave the house without my bag of raw veggies, whether it's snow peas or carrots or cauliflower. So when I get the urge to chew on something (or of course if I actually get hungry!), I have crunchy snacks right at my fingertips. Snow peas may not sound as satisfying as a Snickers bar, but once you change your tastes and form new habits, you'll be very surprised. Our Sugar Savvy Sisters sure were!

"I never thought I'd give up crackers," recalls Bonnie O'Gallagher, 62. "But then I started reaching for cauliflower and hummus. It's just the crunch I'm looking for and it's very satisfying!"

Here's the other thing: You may have no clue that you're actually self-medicating. Our goal is to make you stop and think before it becomes an out-of-control situation. I've worked with people who had no idea they were diving into a jar of peanut butter every evening because they were frustrated with their dead-end job; they just knew they were unhappy. Others set up a nightly ménage a trois with Ben & Jerry because they were lonely. We promise we're going to help you change what you want and that means changing how you respond to your trigger feelings as well as changing those taste buds and sugar cravings. The following quizzes examine your current emotional state regarding your work, personal life, relationships, and financial situation and offer suggestions for dealing with these potential emotional-eating land mines. Answer HONESTLY!

On the Job   TRUE OR FALSE

1 On Friday afternoons, when I leave work, I'm so relieved.
Thank God that the week is finally over.   T   F

2 My boss/supervisor is overbearing and critical.
It drives me crazy.   T   F

3 I always feel like I can't catch up with everything I need
to do.   T   F

4 I'm trapped. I'd leave this job in a minute if I didn't need
the money.   T   F

5 My job is okay; it's the gossip and office politics that get
me down.   T   F

6 My job is going nowhere and I'm so bored with it, but I'm
not qualified for anything else.   T   F

If you answered *True* to one or more of those statements—especially if it's more than three—your work life could be a major food trigger. Being constantly swamped, getting mired in the negativity of co-workers, and feeling trapped for 8 or 9 or more hours a day is a BIG TIME stress and one that can send you straight to the vending machine for a sugar fix!

So what do you do if work leaves you so drained and miserable that you've got a pit in your stomach (waiting to be filled with a sugar-fueled all-you-can-eat brunch!) because tomorrow is Monday? First, remember that eating CRAP will just make you feel worse, physically and mentally. ALWAYS be prepared with Sugar Savvy food on hand. And practice your affirmations throughout the day, repeating them every time you feel frustrated. Take breaks as often as possible. You don't have to run out to the gym (though that can help, too!); simply stand up and stretch, do a few

JOB GOT YOU DOWN?

Repeat these to yourself
at least 3 times a day!

I am happy! I am healthy!
I am the master of my fate.
It is never too late!

I am happy! I am healthy!
I am smart and competent!

I am happy! I am healthy!
I can be anything I want
to be!

squats, and take a quick lap around the hall. Energize your workspace! Being stuck behind four drab brown cubicle walls day in and out is enough to make anyone reach for a Snickers and a soda! Go to the dollar store and get some glitter. Get some shiny flower vases and cut flowers to put in your workspace. You'll be amazed at how quickly your mood improves!

If work is a constant source of sadness, and sugar cravings, start plotting an escape route. Update your resume. Check out job opportunities on career sites. Get out and interview for positions even if they're not perfect. The act of seeking and thinking about what you want to do will make you feel less trapped and will eventually lead to a better place!

Or maybe you actually LIKE your job but still find that it's a constant source of stress and sugar binges. In that case you need better tools for coping and staying centered. I swear by Moving Affirmations (pages 220–225). These are like moving meditation with a stress-blasting endorphin kick! It is IMPOSSIBLE to feel stressed out after you perform them!

"You" Time   TRUE OR FALSE

1 My only moments of "private" time are when I take a shower, go to the bathroom, or get a haircut or manicure.   T   F

2 My husband and I haven't had a night alone since the kids were born.   T   F

3 My elderly parent(s) want(s) to live with me. I'm not sure I can handle it. But I can't say no.   T   F

4 Dating is out of the question for me. As a single mom, I work all day and the only time I see my kids is at night and on the weekends.   T   F

5 My work hours are so long, it's not even a question of balancing a personal and professional life. I don't have a personal life!   T   F

6 My work hours aren't so terrible. But I'm tied to my iPhone/Blackberry 24/7. My boss expects me to be at his/her beck and call evenings and even weekends.   T   F

If you answered *True* to any of these statements (or identified with one or more of them even if they weren't exactly representative of your situation), chances are good you're searching for a sugar high to balance out the energy lows you're feeling by having no time for yourself!

> ## Do NOT feel guilty about buying yourself some time to be alone!

I can tell you one thing right now: **You are not alone.** Everyone I talk to today has more on their plate than they can handle. The first step is waking up to the fact that you DO feel overwhelmed. Then identify what's making you feel that way and think up some amazing, fun, exciting, noneating solutions.

If the only time you have time for yourself is when you're getting your hair or nails done, book a regular appointment and hold on to it with your life! Do NOT feel guilty about buying yourself some time to be alone and hear yourself think! If you can't afford that as often as you'd like, get together with some friends so you **all** can get some much-needed time to get out and have some fun and enjoy some vital "me" time. If you're a mom, arrange to trade off child care with other moms so you can do this. Remember, you are the most important person in your life. Just like when the flight attendant explains that in an emergency you need to put on your own oxygen mask FIRST before helping your kids, you have to take care of your own self before you can help others!

Finally, and I think most importantly, **be gentle** with yourself! Women so often think everything has to be done and it needs to be done perfectly! The dishes always need to be clean and away, the

NO TIME FOR YOU?

Remind yourself daily that you are worth taking time to take care of!

I am happy! I am healthy!
I deserve the time to let myself shine!

I am happy! I am healthy!
Time for ME is a necessity!

I am happy! I am healthy!
I am my first priority!

laundry folded, the house tidy. ***Let go of some of it.*** If the laundry goes undone for a day or even a week, so what? Really. So what? If that's what's standing between you and a Zumba class or a relaxing bath—let it go for a day! Also, you don't need to be the one who always says yes when people ask for volunteers! Say NO once in a while. It feels good! You're not a bad mother, daughter, wife, girlfriend, or friend if you acknowledge that you need a little break.

You will have more energy for everyone else when you take better care of yourself—and that includes eating the Sugar Savvy way. "I'm so much happier now," says Arlene Pineda, 58. "Following this plan has given me the confidence and the energy to make a shift in my life. I'm taking care of myself and I feel better and happier every single day. I'm important and now I know I can treat myself as a priority."

Relationships   TRUE OR FALSE

1. Every time I talk to my husband (boyfriend/significant other), I feel completely misunderstood. We argue constantly.   T   F

2. We don't have anything to say to each other anymore— besides talking about the kids.   T   F

3. We always do the same things and go the same places (when we go anywhere). I'm bored.   T   F

4. I can't remember the last time I had great sex . . . or sex at all, for that matter.   T   F

5. Everywhere I go, I see happy couples. I'm tired of being alone.   T   F

6. How could anyone be interested in someone like me? I even turn myself off.   T   F

Any of those statements ring true? Realize that problems in relationships are one of the biggest emotional triggers out there! Here's the thing, however: ***First and foremost, you must love yourself!*** That's what these affirmations are all about—getting you to a place where you truly love yourself, want the best for yourself, and are willing to do the hard work that it takes to GET the best for yourself. It's a place where you're not stuffing down your feelings with cheesecake, but dealing with them in a powerful, self-loving, and caring way.

Speaking of power and self-love and empowerment, this is the perfect place to address an issue I think is extremely important for women—masturbation. Yep. I just said that. Far too often, I see women caught up in bad relationships for sex—and it's not even good sex! Look, I'm going to be blunt. Orgasms are a wonderful endorphin rush, and they're energizing! If I had my way, every woman would start the day with some mental, spiritual, AND physical self-love! Because loving yourself is the first step to being able to have a loving relationship. Enough said!

Finally, I'll admit that relationships can be especially tricky even for those of us who have plenty of self-love because they're not completely under our own control. There's another person and their feelings to deal with as well, and sometimes it sure feels easier to deny there's anything wrong than to work it out! But now that you've identified the problem or problems, it's time to **talk it out, work it out—or get out!** All the affirmations and self-love in the world still won't change anyone else's behavior, but they WILL change how you respond to it. And it won't be with FOOD.

"This plan has forced me to wake up to ALL the

> ## Affirmations will get you to a place where **you truly love yourself.**

LONELY?

These are biggies, sweetie! You deserve to be with someone who loves and supports you as much as YOU do!

I am happy! I am healthy! I am beautiful and smart with a loving heart!

I am happy! I am healthy! I love myself! I care for myself!

I am happy! I am healthy! I am the best! I deserve the best!!

(continued on page 64)

Sugar Savvy Sisters in Their Own Words

Megan Johnston, Age 22

Went from **exhausted to energized**

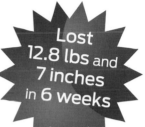

Lost 12.8 lbs and 7 inches in 6 weeks

"I'm very active. I dance and run and do P90X workouts but I still felt down, tired, and heavy. Sugar Savvy intrigued me because I thought it was a great idea to eliminate foods and additives that can take away your energy. I'd also fallen into some bad eating habits of just grabbing anything on the go and eating too much bread and pasta. So I wanted to improve my eating habits in general.

"Giving up bread and pasta was definitely hard the first week. I'm a babysitter, so it was also hard not eating all those kid's foods like Goldfish and mac and cheese. I needed to make myself prepare the night before and have all my foods with me so I wouldn't end up grabbing and eating whatever was available.

"It really worked. My taste buds really have changed and I want healthy foods instead of crap foods. I feel more energized and full of life. Not only are my clothes fitting nicer, even a bit baggy, but also my self-esteem is higher.

"You have to be prepared to change the way you live, because this really is an entirely different way of living, not just some diet. The most powerful part is being able to look at foods and make healthy decisions. I now know exactly what I am putting into my body and how it is helping me be my best. It's a commitment and work at first, but it is very worth it."

(continued from page 62)

negative influences in my life—not just Oreo cookies and cakes!" says Sugar Savvy Sister Cheryl Lee. "When I started this program, I had been dating a man for about a year, knowing he really wasn't the most positive influence in my life. I finally realized I had to put me first and I have finally moved on. I have become more secure in my own self. That's a huge step forward in everything in life!"

Money, Honey   TRUE OR FALSE

		T	F
1	At the end of the month, if it weren't for my overdraft protection, I'd probably be evicted.	T	F
2	No matter how hard we work, we just can't seem to get ahead.	T	F
3	If I leave the house, I don't come home without a shopping bag—or two.	T	F
4	I don't know where my money goes, but cash seems to fly out of my bank account.	T	F
5	My kids want a lot of things we just can't afford, but I buy them anyway.	T	F
6	If my partner or I lost our job, we'd be in BIG trouble in a hurry.	T	F

Any of these sound familiar? If even just one or two of these rang true, you likely have at least a little financial angst. Trust me, you're not alone! Money is always a stress—and no matter how much you make, there never seems to be enough! In tough economic times, it can be extremely worrisome wondering where the next paycheck will come from and how far it will go.

Money is also at the root of a lot of people's terrible eating habits. I hear it all the time: "But Voltage, I can't afford healthy food!" people will say as they make excuses for grabbing a bunch of dollar meals or other fast-food junk. And I always say the same thing: You can't afford to NOT eat healthy food! How much is your diabetes medicine? How much are heart meds? How much are the hospital and doctor bills when (not if) you end up there with clogged arteries and out-of-control blood sugar levels? What's the cost of feeling depressed all the time? What's the cost of leading an unhappy life because you're literally being weighed down not just by worry, but also by all that extra weight you're carrying around because the food you eat is poisoning you? What's the cost of carrying the burden of unwanted extra weight? *Really think about it!*

Healthy food does not have to be expensive food. Beans are very affordable. Check the stores for specials on their fresh produce and meats and fish. Smart shoppers can save a bundle and still eat Sugar Savvy! Since retiring from my private practice, I've watched the people I work with in my not-for-profit programs manage to eat amazing, affordable Sugar Savvy foods every single day! And believe me, plenty of these people have fallen on their share of tough economic times!

Money issues also can and SHOULD be dealt with. If your money issues are literally eating you alive—and sending you to the fridge to eat yourself into a stupor—you *must* deal with them. If you're in truly dire straits, call a credit counselor. There are many ways available to help you avoid financial ruin! Just pick up the phone and I guarantee you'll feel a weight lifted immediately!

If your situation is less serious, but you worry about finances, remember that you are in control here. Are you buying things to fill a void inside? Like overeating, that's a temporary solution that will backfire and leave

WORRIED ABOUT MONEY?

We've all got money woes. Some positive self-talk can give you a free lift!

I am happy! I am healthy! Love and health are my wealth!

I am happy! I am healthy! My future is bright with possibility!

I am happy! I am healthy! All is mine by divine design!

Yes, You CAN Afford to Eat Sugar Savvy!

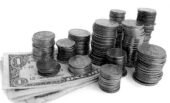 "But Voltage, I can't afford to eat fresh fruits and vegetables. This food is too expensive!" I hear it time and time again. People are used to dollar burgers and fries, shakes, and sandwiches for under five bucks. Yes, buying real food can cost more, but not as much as you might think, especially when you consider real food will help you avoid blood pressure pills, insulin for diabetes, and a mound of medical expenses! But even when you DON'T take those economic benefits into account, you can STILL afford to eat Sugar Savvy *because if you're like most Americans you're spending far more on junk food than you realize!*

According to a new report released by the Economic Research Service of the US Department of Agriculture, Americans spend 17 percent of their food shopping dollars on processed grain foods like pastas and bagels (which is three times what the USDA recommends) and blow about 14 percent of their food budget—about $103 a month—on sweets! (The USDA actually advises that we spend less than 1 percent of our food dollars on sugary sweets.) Meanwhile, we pinch our pennies and dole out a measly, very sad 0.5 percent of our grocery money on green leafy vegetables and just 4 percent on fruit. Guess what? We should be spending about 30 percent of our food dollars on those Sugar Savvy foods instead.

It's simple math, folks! Take the money that you're spending each week on processed grains, pastas, breads, and sweet empty calorie foods that are leaving you run-down, overweight, and sick, and spend the same cash on Sugar Savvy foods that will leave you slim, energized, and looking and feeling terrific! It makes good cents—and sense.

Remember, you are the best. You deserve the best. And to get the best, you have to get your power back. Speak with your dollars. Tell the food manufacturers you don't want their CRAP. Use your spending power to get the best and be the best! Our Sugar Savvy Sisters were pleasantly surprised that they really weren't paying more; they were just buying different foods. Once you try our specially designed meal plan, you'll learn just how simple, affordable, and—most importantly—delicious eating Sugar Savvy can be!

you feeling worse than you did every single time! Say your affirmations. Make yourself happy without plunking down your plastic for yet another pair of shoes you don't really need. Reel in the excess by keeping a spending diary just as you're keeping your food diary. It's really eye-opening and will help you get your spending in check! Most of us don't need more crap, whether it's food or things.

The good news is that once you start, you may find that becoming Sugar Savvy actually SAVES you money so it takes away some of the financial stress in your life. "We discovered that making our own food at home was much less expensive than eating out all the time like we were—and obviously the food is *so* much better for you," says Sugar Savvy Sister Jackie Georgantzas. "The ingredients are simple and affordable. You can make two or three meals for what you might spend on one eating out."

Jealousy Issues   TRUE OR FALSE

1 I spend a lot of time on Facebook and other social media sites. Everyone seems to be living a better, more exciting life than I am.   T   F

2 I hate shopping with my friends because they can afford to spend more than I can.   T   F

3 I sometimes find myself saying mean things about my friends behind their backs even though I feel bad about it later.   T   F

4 I worry that my husband/boyfriend will leave me for someone prettier and younger.   T   F

5 I feel ripped off in life. Everyone seems to have it better than I do.   T   F

6 I'm always waiting for my life to begin. Once I lose 30 pounds or fall into some money, I'll finally be able to live the life I want.   T   F

FEELING JEALOUS?

Kick jealousy to the curb and be the star of your own wonderful life right now! Repeat after me:

I am happy! I am healthy!
My life is full and complete!

I am happy! I am healthy!
My inner light is shining bright!

I am happy! I am healthy!
All I need is within me now!

People use food highs to fill many voids and to lift themselves out (at least temporarily!) of many lows. Jealousy in life can be a **big black hole!** If you answered True to one or more of the questions above, jealousy is definitely one of your trigger feelings. Life is too short to always be looking around at what everyone else has got without appreciating all the wonderful things around you!

I've worked with the most beautiful, famous women in the world. We're talking women with long, perfect legs up to their necks, flowing shiny locks, and impeccable skin, who are perfectly miserable! They look around themselves and never feel like they're pretty enough or thin enough or successful enough. What a waste!!! They should be living large and enjoying life beyond their wildest dreams and all they can think about is what they imagine they don't have.

To be Sugar Savvy is about changing what you want, right? Well, that means in your life, too! Unhappy about how your weight compares to other people's? You can't control their weight, but you can decide that you are worthy and beautiful and start working toward changing your weight right now. There is no room in the Sugar Savvy mind-set for self-pity! There is no room for "Woe is me; if you had my life, you'd eat CRAP, too." Everyone has hard times and burdens to bear. Sugar Savvy living means you assume an attitude of gratitude! Because the most important thing is that you are *you* and you are here and alive and able to take this journey. When you start really living the Sugar Savvy life and loving yourself and brimming with energy, trust me, you'll be so happy being you, you won't remember what you were so jealous of anymore.

TRIGGER SITUATIONS

Finally, along with trigger foods and emotional triggers, there are trigger places and situations. I'm sure you can think of a few obvious ones—parties (we'll talk more about alcohol later!), movies, happy hours, dinner dates, family gatherings, and sporting events, just to name a few!

Ask yourself very honestly: Are there places where you always overeat? Is it that the foods in those places are so unbelievably delectable that you just can't help eating everything in sight? Butter-sopped stale popcorn and hotdogs and chicken wings and chips and dips? I DON'T THINK SO, FOLKS! Is it because everyone else is pigging out and you don't want to look like a party pooper? If you look more closely (especially at some of the fitter-looking men and women), you'll notice that not *everyone* is gorging. There are likely more than a few smart folks clutching sparkling water and plates of cut veggies and fruit. I'm guessing this social overeating is just a habit. Think about it: Are you even hungry when you go to these places? Or are you just eating because food is there and that's what you do? Is that what you really want? **No.**

I'm not going to ask you to live the life of a hermit, of course! As you develop your new relationship with food and become Sugar Savvy, you'll be able to enjoy a full social life without worrying or obsessing over food—talk about liberating, huh? This is where all your affirmation work comes in. As you're walking into your trigger environment, whip out this affirmation and repeat it over and over, burning it into your brain:

> ∗ I am happy, I am healthy,
> I can eat what I want because I've changed what I want!

Now, look around the room with Sugar Savvy eyes and Sugar Savvy wisdom and Sugar Savvy confidence. I will bet you those French fries that smelled so irresistible now look greasy and gross. That pizza oozing oil under the heat lamps? Ugh! The giant, flour-filled cookies wrapped in

(continued on page 72)

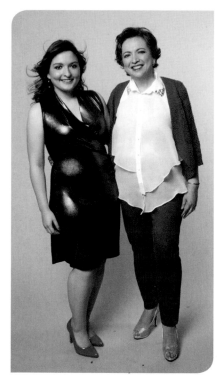

Arlene Pineda, Age 58

Jackie Georgantzas, Age 20

This **mother and daughter got closer** as they made a joint effort to **kick their sugar habit** and eat Sugar Savvy meals.

Jackie and her mom Arlene did the Sugar Savvy plan as a team, determined to work together toward permanent lifestyle changes. Both were self-proclaimed sugar junkies who often used food as therapy. As Arlene put it, "I turn to breads, cakes, and chocolates for energy and to lift my mood." But life had thrown them a curveball in the form of cancer that inspired them to change for good.

Together lost 11.6 lbs and 6 inches in 6 weeks!

"I had a tumor removed from my pancreas," explained Arlene. "Now I have a smaller pancreas that will work harder. I don't want diabetes from my bad eating habits." Her daughter's health wasn't in immediate jeopardy, but she was weary of the weight-loss roller coaster. "My weight has gone up and down and up and down because I've never really changed my eating habits. I've had that 'you can't have that' diet mentality, which always left me feeling deprived,

> "We're doing this as a family so we are healthier and can pass it along to our future family."

so I'd go right back to my old ways," says Jackie.

For them, education was everything. "The Sugar Savvy solution doesn't just say, 'You can't eat this or that.' This tells you what is really going on with those foods and why you're craving them," says Arlene. "It gives you a real message to work with—about loving yourself and making the best decisions for your life. Life is precious. Be grateful and take care of yourself."

In that vein, Jackie and Arlene have made cooking at home a priority. "We eat out far less," says Jackie. "We go to the supermarket each week and buy our produce and cut it up right away so it's easy to use. When we do go out, we ask lots of questions and we always ask for vegetables.

"At first I struggled to drink enough water, but I kept at it, and now it's a habit. I learned that all grains—even the healthy ones like brown rice—are trigger foods for me," says Jackie. "So I focus on eating other carbohydrates, like vegetables. I don't crave sweets or diet sodas, which I drank constantly, anymore. I used to be very tired in the morning and could barely think about breakfast. Now I have a Vital Veggie breakfast every morning. And I have lots of energy and mental clarity. It's really cool."

After 8 months of eating Sugar Savvy, Jackie has dropped a total of 14.8 pounds and Arlene 19.2 pounds—reaching her goal weight!

Arlene's favorite affirmation: I am happy! I am healthy! I am the best! And I deserve the best!

Jackie's favorite affirmation: I am happy! I am healthy! I'm beautiful, strong, and smart!

Sweet Dreams!

The Sugar Savvy solution is about complete, positive lifestyle change. Well, there's one enormous part of your life we haven't talked about that is *critical* for your Sugar Savvy success: SLEEP!

They don't call it "beauty sleep" for nothing! While you sleep, your body repairs, regenerates, and recharges for another day. Your body NEEDS between 7 and 9 hours of sleep a night to look and perform its best! Shortchanging your sleep not only makes you look tired and run-down, but research shows that just one sleepless night interferes with your body's ability to use insulin and manage your blood sugar levels. Shortchange your sleep by getting less than 6 hours a night, and you're three times more likely to have high blood sugar levels. Too little sleep also wreaks havoc on your hormones (especially your stress hormones like cortisol), which makes you more prone to overeat, store fat, and gain weight.

In fact, study after study shows that the less sleep you get, the more likely you are to be overweight. In one landmark study 68,000 women, those who slept only 5 hours a night were 32 percent more likely to gain 33 pounds or more over 16 years compared to the women who got a solid 7 hours of shut-eye a night!

The good news is that by following the Sugar Savvy plan, you'll be eating healthier, more nourishing food, moving your body every day, and blasting stress with positive affirmations—all of which promote quality sleep.

(continued from page 69)

a body bag (I mean plastic wrap)? You honest-to-God do not want that CRAP anymore. Are you really hungry? If not, walk right on by and enjoy your party, ball game, or social event. If yes, look for a lively and energizing fresh fruit cup or satisfying crunchy crudités? I also recommend having a Sugar Savvy snack before going out if you don't know what food will be on hand. You'll be better able to make good decisions and pass by the junk. Once you've changed your taste buds and decided to never let yourself get too hungry and always be fully prepared, there's no going back, honey!

YOUR FRESH START BEGINS NOW!

Now that you're wide awake to the power that trigger foods and food addiction have had over you, it's time to break the spell! You'll find the full Sugar Savvy meal plan starting on page 150. But right now, before you head to the store to buy your new food supply, I want you to take a look in your pantry. Grab a package of something you normally eat and take a look at the ingredient list. Is it a mile long? Are there things on there that you can't pronounce? ***It's probably not on our plan***. This is about back-to-the-basics, really good, really nutritious, **real old-school food**—or as one of my heroes, Michael Pollan, says, "ones your ancestors would recognize!" And, of course, it's about getting the added sugars that infiltrate our processed foods out!

I bet you haven't even begun to open your eyes (and mouth) to all the delicious possibilities that the world of real food has to offer! Sugar Savvy food isn't boring or tasteless; it tastes amazing! Do you think you hate vegetables? Well, if your only experience with veggies has been with canned, mushed, oversalted, overprocessed vegetables, then I don't blame you, sweetie!

Many of our Sugar Savvy Sisters turned up their noses when they first saw "green drinks" made with spinach or kale. Others were sure they were going to hate anything with broccoli. But then they got a taste of the AMAZING fresh roasted, grilled, or steamed eggplant, squash, peppers, mushrooms, broccoli, spinach, and so forth that are part of the Sugar Savvy plan, and they flipped!

I made a deal with all of them: "You don't have to eat everything I suggest, but you DO have to taste it." I want you to make the same vow to yourself. Even if you've never seen it before or had it before, **try it**. Clear your mind of your preconceived notions about what "something green" is going to taste like. You have no idea until you put it in your mouth! So try it! What's the worst-case scenario? You spit it out. I doubt you will, but you just don't know till you give it a shot. That's what this is all about!

Remember, the number one goal of this entire plan is ***changing what you want***. As you leave behind all those trigger foods, you will start to want all sorts of new, fresh foods. And the more of these foods you try through our plan, the more you'll want and the less you'll even think about all that tired old processed stuff you don't want anymore! That is truly the Sugar Savvy solution!

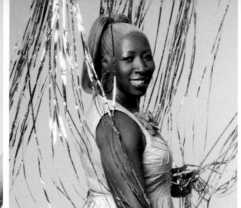
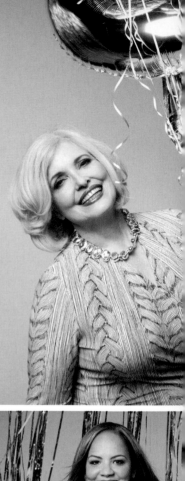
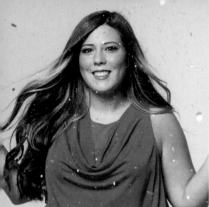
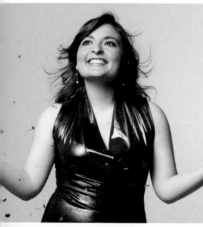
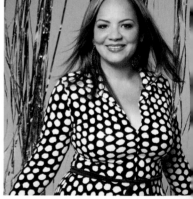
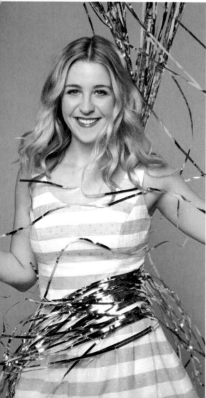
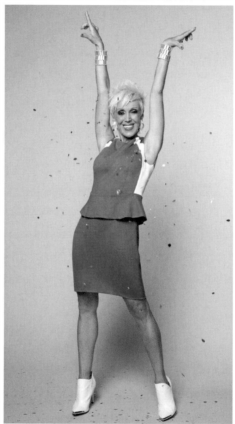
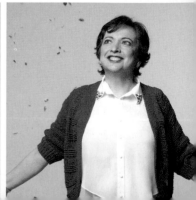
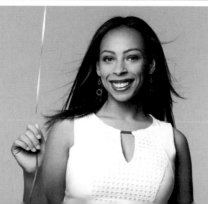

PART 2

THE SUGAR SAVVY SOLUTION:

6 WEEKS TO FIT, FABULOUS, AND FIERCE!

How many times have you thought, "If only I wasn't so heavy (or tired, or stressed out)?" THIS IS YOUR CHANCE! The Sugar Savvy solution is your roadmap to living more fully than you thought possible! As I mentioned in Chapter 1, my five STAR points are an essential foundation to CHANGE WHAT YOU WANT and create your new normal:

- Get hydrated.
- Eat Sugar Savvy approved.
- Move your body.
- Announce your affirmations loudly and proudly!
- Be kind and assume an attitude of gratitude and forgiveness.

In this section, you'll find a step-by-step guide to incorporating each of these points into your life—and transforming your body, mind, and spirit! Over the next 6 weeks, you'll get much more than a diet and exercise program (you'll find details on those in Part 3 for easy reference); you'll get a jump start to creating your Sugar Savvy life and sticking to it, week by week.

CHAPTER 4

WEEK 1: JUMP-START YOUR SUGAR SAVVY LIFE

Cleanse your mind, your home, and your palate.

"I used to hoard food—chips, pretzels, Doritos, snack food of all sorts— so I knew it would be there, in my desk drawer or wherever I needed it when a craving hit. At 2 p.m. I could just eat a whole bag of salt and vinegar chips. I'd polish off half a box of sourdough pretzels before bed, so I would wake up feeling sick. I was out of control and setting myself up for failure at every turn."

—PERRI O. BLUMBERG, 24,
WHO LOST **11.2 POUNDS** IN **6 WEEKS**

SUGAR SLEUTHING

During the next week, I would like you to go through your kitchen—the fridge, the cupboards, and the pantry—and read labels. Write down how many sugar grams are in the things you eat. Don't forget to include beverages— sodas, teas, juices, everything! Take a few days for this exercise. If you frequent fast-food places and restaurant chains, quickly look up your favorite go-to meals online and write down the amount of sugar in those as well.

It's important that you really look at what you **have** been eating so you can **truly** understand how important it is that we change that! Take the time to do the sugar shocker exercises (see page 23) with all the processed foods you eat on a regular basis (you don't have to do this with fresh food, like produce and lean meats). Hands down, every Sugar Savvy Sister told us that this exercise was the single biggest thing that inspired her to really, finally change! **So do it!**

Another exercise that may shock you? Record how many sugar grams you consume this week on the following chart:

	Breakfast	Lunch	Dinner	Snacks	TOTAL
Day 1					
Day 2					
Day 3					
Day 4					
Day 5					
Day 6					
Day 7					

Remember, the Sugar Savvy goal is no more than 24 grams of added sugar in 24 hours. If you take on the challenge of the Soupalicious Palate Cleanse this week, that won't be a problem. If not, this may inspire you to try it!

BRAIN WASHING

This week I also want you to do a Sugar Savvy "brain wash" to undo all the pervasive negative and UNTRUE messages and lies, lies, lies you've been subjected to about willpower and what a loser you are because you can't control your eating. Like most women I know, you probably run negative messages through your mind from morning till night! Wash all those negative thoughts out of that brain! If you haven't already, I want you to start practicing your positive affirmations every single day. Starting this week, I want you to write them down in the morning and at night. Experience has taught me that five is the magic number. So each morning, I want you to write five times:

* I am happy!

* I am healthy!

* I am _____!

(Fill in the blank with a positive, uplifting statement about yourself. For example, "I am strong and powerful and nothing can stop me now!" Borrow from the ones sprinkled throughout the book or on page 123 if you need to.)

Then, before you go to bed, write them five more times. You'll find that the more you write them, the more you'll mean them—that's how creating new tapes in your brain works! Trust me, **words are powerful.**

THE SOUPALICIOUS PALATE CLEANSE

Finally, and VERY IMPORTANTLY this week, I would like you to "wipe the slate clean" and reset your taste buds with the 3- to 5-day Soupalicious Palate Cleanse. As you know, there was a point in my life when I was an out-of-control sugar junkie. I had shaken a drug problem and dealt with alcoholism, but I couldn't resist cookies and doughnuts. One bite and the

Victim No More!

You've heard me say many, many times that it's not your fault that one bite of trigger foods turns into a full-on binge. This is by design. The food companies want you to eat and eat and eat, and they manipulate their foods to trigger all the right brain chemicals that will keep you coming back for more. However, it is VERY important to realize that this does NOT make you a victim!

You are not powerless! Far from it. Remember, when the Big Food companies tell us, "We only sell what people want," they're right. So it's time to CHANGE WHAT YOU want and tell them loudly and proudly that you want better choices than the CRAP they're selling.

box was gone—sometimes two boxes! Did I ever crave carrots and celery and turnips and greens? Yeah, right! Only if someone could have managed to deep-fry and sugarcoat them! The only "carats" I was interested in were in my diamond rings!

Recognizing the pattern of addiction, I realized that my chronic sugar consumption was a serious brain chemistry problem. I also realized that my taste buds had been **beaten to death!** Remember, a steady diet of sugar-laden processed foods strips your taste buds of their ability to taste anything but those CRAP (Calories Robbed at Processing) processed foods. So I could no longer recognize real food!

I needed to do something radical to change my tastes and reboot my brain! I needed to revive my deadened buds and learn to want, love, and yes, CRAVE vegetables and fruits and all the amazing foods that have been put on this planet for me to enjoy! That's when I created the Soupalicious Palate Cleanse.

The Palate Cleanse is just what it sounds like—a way for you to scrub your palate clean from the dulling effects of a constant assault of foods that are too sweet and too salty and reset it so it's open to a fresh Sugar Savvy beginning. In his new book *Disease Proof,* Dr. David Katz, director of the Yale Prevention Research Center, devotes a chapter to what he calls "Taste Bud Rehab"—which I love, because it gives a medical nod to the food addiction problem I've been preaching about for three decades! Guess what he recommends? You got it—eliminating hidden sugar and salt, then re-educating and rehabilitating your taste buds.

The Palate Cleanse is a complete system to do just that! Combined with the rest of my Sugar Savvy plan, it also rewires your brain, short-circuiting sugar cravings. Even better, you're going to supercharge your body with energy-boosting and health-promoting nutrition in a way that it may have never been charged before! You're going to feel Fit, Fab, and Fierce from the inside out, with **abundant energy!**

Change What You Want—FAST

The Soupalicious Palate Cleanse is the single most powerful way to jump-start a healthy way of eating (by making a big statement that you're really ready to make a change). It is also a program you can return to if trigger foods become a problem again or you slide off track and the weight creeps back on. To this day, I do the cleanse every few months to stay in tip-top shape.

> A steady diet of sugar-laden foods **strips your taste buds** of their ability to taste anything but CRAP processed foods.

How fast does the Palate Cleanse work? Just ask Arlene, who in our first meeting told me how sugar control was a constant struggle. "I need to see if I'm capable of breaking my habit of eating sweets, especially when I am tired. I always reach for comfort foods like cakes, breads, and chocolates," she lamented. "I need to understand what is holding me back from enjoying healthy eating and to make a permanent change."

Just 5 days later, she sent me a message singing the praises of newfound love of all the whole, fresh, wonderful foods she was enjoying as part of her Palate Cleanse. "The soup is amazing. I put in a sweet potato, kale, garlic, beets, carrots, white mushrooms, one leek, some onion, turnip, butternut squash, and zucchini. It's wonderful! We added some black beans, amino acids, and coconut oil, too. It's so-o-o good!"

Though it's not the point, Arlene also lost 3½ pounds *just that week*. And Megan Johnston, who was tired of feeling weighed down by bread and pasta, dropped nearly a full dress size, losing 8½ pounds. Others lost 1 to 8 pounds—all from the cleanse alone!

And listen up, because this is the important part: **These women weren't hungry.** They weren't walking around feeling deprived. They weren't starving themselves. They were NOURISHING themselves. This cleanse is so nutritious and hydrating that people who go on it are generally shocked that they're no longer hungry all the time!

> Our bodies never really get all the nutrients they need. **So we keep eating** while never actually nourishing ourselves!

Sugar Savvy Sister Nancy Barthold in particular was amazed by that revelation. She told me during our initial meeting how she often felt helpless against her overeating. She would just eat and eat and eat all evening long. Once she started the cleanse, that stopped. More importantly, the DESIRE to hunt for food stopped. "I found it to be much easier than I expected," she says. "By the end of the third day, I was ready for a 'regular meal,' but I really appreciated that. The cleanse made me really acknowledge true hunger as opposed to just wanting to eat."

I am firmly convinced that much of our overeating is due to poor nutrition "thanks" to processed foods. Our bodies never really get all the nutrients they need, so we keep searching and eating and searching and eating, gaining unwanted pounds, while never actually nourishing ourselves!

Over time, you'll actually develop an aversion to the nutritionally barren, overprocessed foods you thought you loved. In *Disease Proof,* Dr. David Katz reports that women participating in the landmark Iowa Women's Health Study (in progress since the 1980s!) who started eating a lower-fat, plant-based diet during the study eventually stopped eating junk food, not because they were supposed to, but because they no longer liked it! That's what this is about: *eating what you want because you have changed what you want*!

Reset Your Taste Buds with Soupalicious Soup

Time to get started! Let me repeat, the intention of the cleanse is to change your eating behaviors (like the constant need to munch or put fork to mouth) and give your palate a break from sugar and its evil sidekicks. It is NOT a fast. It is NOT about eating as little as possible. It is NOT about starving yourself or seeing how little you can eat or drinking just water and lemon juice. It is about

Back to Nature!

I read a fascinating article in *The Telegraph* (a British paper that publishes online) about how farmers there are fearful that the population there (like here) has desensitized their taste buds with sugar- and salt-laden processed foods! Fiona Reynolds, director of the National Trust, says, "Taste [for fresh foods] is something we're losing, because too many of our meals are packed with additives and flavorings."

THAT is how powerful the processed food industry is. It's robbing whole nations of their taste for **real, wholesome natural foods**! It's time to take our power back! And it starts with the Palate Cleanse. Your taste buds CAN be revitalized. Your brain CAN start to crave different flavors and real foods. Your body will REALLY appreciate the nourishment. You will feel Fit, Fabulous, and Fierce. You just have to take this very important first step!

packing as much nutrition into your body as you can to get yourself feeling Fit, Fab, and Fierce!

The way to do this is very simple: soup!—or, as I say, Soupalicious! I have been preaching the praises of soup for decades. For this plan, I asked my friend Jessica Issler, a registered dietitian, to help me make the Soupalicious Soup as hearty, healthy, and Sugar Savvy as possible! There is no better way to jam-pack nutrition into your system than this. It's bursting with veggies—far more than the measly one or two servings a day you get on the standard American diet (SAD)—which provide filling fiber, healthy carbohydrates, and anti-aging antioxidants. Plus, the beans add lean protein and coconut oil (my fave!) gives you a dose of good-for-you fats.

Make a batch of Soupalicious Soup from the recipe at right. **Eat 1 to 2 cups every 2 hours or so to get nutrition throughout the day.** That's it! You can wash down your soup with water or chase it with a power-packed green drink (recipe on page 88). Practice the Palate Cleanse for 3 to 5 days.

It may feel monotonous to have nothing but Soupalicious Soup all day, but remember that the point here is to reset your buds to really free yourself from the power of sugar. If you crave a bit of variety, try your Soupalicious Soup different ways. You can have it hot or cold. Or you can experiment with different combinations of veggies and spices (especially if you choose to make smaller batches). You can even try it chunky, rather than pureed, though I STRONGLY RECOMMEND pureeing because I really want you to commit to changing your behavior and breaking bad patterns, by giving you a break from CHEWING in the way you normally do. Plus, I have found that this not only allows you to get maximum nutrition—you can get LOTS of veggies into a pureed soup!—but it also seems to make the soup easier to digest.

The first time you do the Palate Cleanse, you may feel a little headache-y or low in energy for the first couple of days. (I recommend that you start it on a weekend, or at a time when you're not super-busy.) This is a detox, after all! But if you stick with it, any discomfort should soon disappear. And, because the Palate Cleanse frees you from the constant "food hunt," you have that much more energy to focus on other areas of your life. "It was way easier than I expected," says Perri O. Blumberg, who, though not overweight, was a serious sugar addict. "I was full all the time, so I wasn't preoccupied with hunting down cookies or snacks."

It takes a bit of effort, but remember: Your reward is losing up to a pound a day while you kick your food addiction to the curb! This may seem like **shock therapy,** and in fact, it is. But sometimes that's exactly what the doctor ordered!

(continued on page 88)

THE SOUPALICIOUS PALATE CLEANSE

2¼ cups dried beans (such as white beans, navy beans, black beans), soaked overnight and sorted to remove any debris

12 cups water, divided

⅓ cup coconut oil or olive oil

2 large sweet potatoes (about 5" long), peeled and chopped

5 to 6 cups chopped fresh nonstarchy vegetables (try carrots, celery, beets, mushrooms, zucchini, summer squash, and leafy greens such as kale, Swiss chard, or spinach)—no canned veggies!

Herbs and spices to taste (such as 4–6 cloves garlic, 1–2 tablespoons fresh basil, rosemary, or thyme, a pinch of ground red pepper or onion powder, etc.)

❶ Rinse the soaked beans thoroughly before cooking. In a large pot over high heat, place the beans and 6 cups of the water. Bring to a boil, then reduce the heat and simmer for about an hour, or until beans are tender.

❷ Add the oil, spices, sweet potatoes, and vegetables and remaining 6 cups of water to the pot and simmer for an additional 30 minutes, or until the vegetables are tender.

❸ Puree, either in a blender or using an immersion blender. **Eat 1 to 2 cups every 2 hours or so.**

This recipe makes enough soup for 2 days. Repeat as desired for up to 5 days. During the cleanse, it is important not to include any foods containing sugar. If you feel dizzy or light-headed, make sure you are drinking enough soup. If you still have problems, stop the cleanse.

Note: I recommend dried beans because canned beans tend to be so high in sodium. If you do opt to use canned beans, choose no-salt-added organic beans, in BPA-free cans, if possible. You would need four to five 15.5-oz. cans. Soak for 30 minutes and rinse to remove as much sodium as possible.

Note: A significant increase in fiber from the beans and veggies can cause some digestive discomfort. To prevent this, be extra vigilant about getting at least 8 glasses of water per day. Additionally, any change in your dietary patterns can interfere with certain medications, so discuss with your healthcare provider before starting the Palate Cleanse.

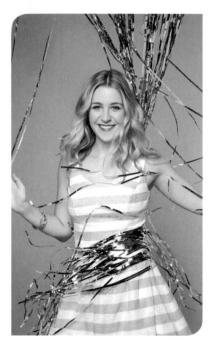

Perri O. Blumberg, Age 24

Feels **free from food addiction** for the first time in her life.

Lost 11.2 lbs and 4¾ inches in 6 weeks!

To look at Perri—fit, active, and lithe—you'd never dream she has a single issue with food, let alone a full-blown addiction. But she did and it was running—and ruining—her life. "I've always struggled with a massive sweet/salty tooth," she explained. "My job as a food editor makes it worse, because it requires me to taste a lot of not-so-healthy foods, and for me there is no such thing as 'just having one.' A single bite of a cookie will keep me coming back until I have devoured the whole box. I also eat out a lot, so bread baskets and desserts were my best friends. Or maybe more like frenemies. I got very tired of waking up bloated and headachy with food hangovers and feeling drained and exhausted all the time.

"It's like food is literally calling to me constantly until I can't resist and I sneak two jumbo candy bars at 3 p.m. I've tried everything to keep the cravings at bay—using different-colored plates, keeping junk food out of my apartment, reading books and magazine articles, meeting with nutritionists—all to

> "Junk food doesn't taste good anymore. It's amazing. I'm free."

no avail. Luckily it doesn't show too much physically, but I have felt the pressure of my food addiction every single day," she says.

Perri's first step to freedom was the Soupalicious Palate Cleanse. "I did it for a week and it really rewired my taste buds. When I poured my usual bowl of Grape-Nuts afterwards, they tasted unbelievably salty. I tried some glazed carrots out at a restaurant and they were gross—so sticky and overly sweet. I got a craving for some sourdough pretzels—an old trigger food—so I thought I'd try one. I had a few bites and that's really all I wanted. If I do crave one of my indulgences, like fried bananas at night, I'll say, 'Okay. You can have it in the morning.' Ninety-nine percent of the time, I no longer want it! And the 1 percent when I do, I have it and I'm done with it! It doesn't consume my thoughts."

Perri lost a few excess pounds, but most importantly, she gained control of her life. "I don't pig out anymore," she says. "I don't go on eating sprees like I used to. I have so much more energy. I feel amazing. I've tried countless eating plans to beat my food obsessions and none of them worked. This did. Now when I think I'm hungry, I first try indulging in relaxing with a magazine, taking a bubble bath, or giving an old friend a call. Afterwards, I realize I wasn't even hungry to begin with! It's amazing what happens when you listen to your body, the way the Sugar Savvy plan rewires you to do!"

> My favorite affirmation: I am happy! I am healthy! I am free from food voices in my head!

(continued from page 84)

Go Green!

If you would like another kind of taste during your cleanse, you can add a green drink. Like the Soupalicious Soup, these leafy green–based drinks are nutritional powerhouses. Wash your Soupalicious Soup and green drinks down with eight glasses of water, and you'll be sparkling with energy and not one bit hungry. This is one of those times I ask you to trust me, and take a leap of faith. Here's how to make a green drink tailored to your very own tastes. (Note: The amounts are just guidelines to get you started. There are no hard-and-fast rules here; adjust as needed to taste. Experiment and have fun!)

HIGH VOLTAGE GREEN DRINK

Fistful or two of leafy greens (such as kale, spinach, or Swiss chard)

Handful of carrots and beets (or other sweet veggie such as tomatoes)

Handful of more subtly flavored vegetable (such as celery, cucumber, sugar snap peas, radishes, or jicama)

Pinch of parsley, fresh cilantro, or fresh ginger

Half a pear or apple (optional)

Water or ice as needed

1 In a blender, place the leafy greens.

2 To cut the bitterness and add a slightly sweet flavor, toss in the carrots and beets or other slightly sweet veggie such as tomatoes.

3 End with a handful of more subtly flavored veggies (your celery, cucumber, sugar snap peas, radish, or jicama).

4 Top it off with a pinch or so of a fresh herb such as parsley, cilantro, or ginger for a little something special! Add half a pear or apple if desired to cut any bitter taste.

5 Blend until thoroughly combined. If it's too thick, add a little water or ice.

As with your Soupalicious Soup, feel free to experiment with different combinations of veggies and herbs, but please always make them yourself. Veggie juices you buy in the store that are bottled and pasteurized may have unwanted sugar or other additives and are not nourishing. Fruit juices (even if squeezed or juiced at home) are really condensed sources of natural sugar and calories, so avoid them, especially at this stage.

Alternatively, you can buy a green drink powder. Look for one with:

- A high ratio of greens to nongreens (most packages show the breakdown in milligrams)
- Minimal fillers, flours, or sweeteners (**no added sugar!**)

Some of my favorite green drink powders are Vibrant Health Green Vibrance, Barlean's Organic Greens, and Amazing Grass Green Superfood. You can generally find these at health food stores like Vitamin Shoppe or online at Amazon and other retailers.

No Starvation

Remember, the goal of the Palate Cleanse is not to starve yourself. In fact, it's exactly the opposite! We're revving up your engine by maximizing the nutrition you're getting. While it's normal to feel a little headache-y at first, if you feel very dizzy or light-headed during the cleanse, it could be a sign that you're not taking in enough nutrition; make sure you're drinking 1 to 2 cups of your Soupalicious Soup every 2 hours or so.

If you do have any problems with the Palate Cleanse, it's okay to skip it. You'll still be able to reset your taste buds by following the Sugar Savvy Meal Plan you'll learn about in the next chapter, and to change your brain by following the rest of the Sugar Savvy solution. But I HIGHLY RECOMMEND IT; *almost all of our Sugar Savvy Sisters did it*, and they swear it was an instrumental part in changing the way they felt about food.

CHAPTER 5

WEEK 2: SLIM DOWN WITH THE SUGAR SAVVY EATING PLAN

Jump right in! Start the Sugar Savvy Meal Plan, hydrate right, and move more often!

"This isn't just another diet. This is a wake-up call—a whole new way of living. After so many years of eating and shopping and living my 'old' way, it was a major adjustment. It took time—it still takes some time—but it's worth it."

—MARVA PHILLIPS, 69,
WHO LOST **10 POUNDS** IN **6 WEEKS**

Sugar Savvy Foundations

This week as we build, continue to:

* Read your labels: Keep sugar sleuthing!
* Say and write your daily affirmations!
* Eat no more than 24 grams of added sugar in 24 hours.

Now that you've seen just how much sugar is in your food and how it's sapping your energy, you're ready to kick it to the curb and replace all those empty calories with real, honest-to-goodness food that fuels your Fit, Fab, and Fierce life!

We'll start by banishing liquid sugar (i.e., soda, juice, and other sugar-sweetened beverages) and replacing it with pure, cleansing H_2O. (Good news: If you did the Palate Cleanse, you've already done this!) Then we'll dive right into making your diet Sugar Savvy by focusing on Sugar Savvy–approved foods and starting the official Sugar Savvy Meal Plan. This week I also want you to start moving your body *every single day!* This may seem like a lot to tackle in 7 days, but I promise it will be easy once you see how all three parts work together to get your **energy up** and your **weight down**! If you find yourself really overwhelmed, though, don't give up—just focus on one thing at a time (i.e., focus on banishing liquid sugar first; then, when you feel comfortable with that, move on to starting the Sugar Savvy Meal Plan, and work at your own pace). And keep writing your affirmations five times in the morning, five times in the evening, and five times when you feel stressed; this will help reinforce your motivation and give you the confidence and energy to do all these new things.

Both approaches can work. But I will say that the Sugar Savvy Sisters who dove in headfirst and did it all in one fell swoop were the most successful. It makes sense. Banishing soda is fantastic, but if you're still drinking juice, eating cookies, and relying on processed CRAP, you aren't freeing yourself to become fully empowered from food addiction. When I was rehabbing from alcohol, they didn't say, "Okay, Kathie [that was before anyone called me Voltage], stop binge drinking, but you can still drink a little light beer." It doesn't really work that way! The same is true for trigger foods. If at all humanly possible, go cold turkey! It may seem harder right now, but it'll be way easier in the long run. I promise you. In order to beat an addiction, you have to acknowledge it for what it is. You can't negotiate with it.

Ready? Let's roll!

BANISH LIQUID SUGAR AND HYDRATE RIGHT

Most Americans guzzle more than 40 gallons of sugar-sweetened beverages (SSBs) every year, but that is NOT, let me repeat NOT, how you stay hydrated!

Why's that? Because proper hydration makes you feel alert and energetic. It helps your muscles work optimally. And it helps your kidneys and liver and other organs flush toxins out of your system so you feel healthy and vibrant. None of that happens if the liquids that you're dumping into your system are loaded with chemicals, artificial colorings, and worst of the worst, *added sugar, which is a poison* when taken in excess.

All you're doing by pouring in gallons of sugar is forcing your organs to labor even harder, making yourself sick (and fat). Forget about being energized—even if you're drinking those so-called "energy drinks." You may soar like a rocket after the first few sips, but then you'll come crashing down like a 2-ton meteor an hour later. So you drink more energy drinks and soda, right? WRONG!

The average 32-ounce soda has as much sugar as a Snickers candy bar or half a bag of Skittles. Puh-leeze! That's liquid candy! And, as you'll remember from our sugar shockers in Chapter 2, fruit juices, flavored teas and lemonades, energy drinks, and enhanced waters may sound healthier

> Proper hydration makes you **feel alert and energetic**, helps your muscles work optimally, and flushes toxins out of your system.

but can have just as much sugar in them. By eliminating regular soda and other flavored nondiet beverages, the average woman can lose *1 pound per week*! You might even save your life. Seriously! Remember, sugary drinks are to blame for the deaths of 180,000 men and women around the world *each year* through conditions like type 2 diabetes and heart disease.

Let's take a cold, hard look at all the ways soda—even the diet kind—can wreck your health. I picked this up from healthychild.com when I started this revolution. It's relevant for ALL of us, no matter our age.

- Soda contains zero nutrients, and it's high in calories and sugar. Studies show a strong link between soda consumption and obesity.

- Phosphorus, a common ingredient in soda, can deplete bones of calcium. Women who drink more soda are more prone to broken bones.

- Studies show a direct link between tooth decay and soda. Not only does the sugar cause cavities, the acids in soda etch off tooth enamel in as little as 20 minutes.

- Drinking a lot of soda every day can lead to blood sugar disorders, including diabetes, and can inhibit proper digestive function.

Enough said! Time to kick soda to the curb!

Drink Eight Glasses of Water Daily

If you want to lose weight, shake the sugar habit, and feel vibrant and alive and bursting with energy, you must be hydrated. That means WATER and lots of it!

Your body is made up of about 60 percent water and you lose this essential fluid every minute of every day as you breathe, digest, and hopefully work up a sweat (remember, we're going to get moving!). It is 100 percent important that you put back every drop. Starting now I want you to **drink eight 8-ounce glasses of water every single day.** That is the non-negotiable Sugar Savvy hydration mantra. Your body needs a minimum of eight glasses of water a day.

Drinking enough water actually helps you combat water retention. Sounds counterintuitive, I know. But think about it. If you're running around in a semi-dehydrated state all the time, your body is going to madly hang on to every single drop, giving you that puffy, unhealthy appearance. When you're properly hydrating, your body gets the message that all systems are operating smoothly and it continues its work of flushing out your system and ridding itself of the excess fluids. Many times when you think you're hungry, sleepy, depressed, and/or irritated, you're actually just dehydrated!

> Many times when you think you're hungry, sleepy, depressed, and/or irritated, **you're actually just dehydrated**!

If your goal is to lose weight, water is a MUST. When you're dehydrated, your body sends out signals that it needs assistance. Many people mistake those thirsty SOS signals for hunger and take in hundreds of extra calories they don't need. They also don't solve the real problem—thirst! Drinking water can act as a powerful appetite suppressant and allow you to cue in to your real hunger. Your body also needs plenty of water for proper digestion, so you can get the most from the foods you eat. You're less susceptible to food cravings when your stomach is full and you're getting all the nutrients you need!

For even more powerful results, drink two 8-ounce glasses of water before every meal—you'll eat less! Virginia Tech researchers found that people who drank 16 ounces of water before sitting down to a meal ate about 85 fewer calories during the meal. Over the course of 12 weeks, the dieters who drank water before every meal lost 5 pounds more than those who didn't.

Your body uses water for fat metabolism, so if you don't drink enough, you don't burn enough fat either. If you're one of those women who is always bemoaning her sluggish metabolism, drink, drink, drink! Water fires up your metabolism, which is a huge bonus since it has zero calories! When German researchers gave 14 men and women two glasses of water, they found that their metabolism began to rise within 10 minutes of their final sip. After 40 minutes, their average calorie-burning rate was 30 percent higher, and it stayed elevated for more than an hour. So drink up!

> German researchers found that metabolism rises **within 10 minutes** of drinking water.

You won't just feel better, you'll also look better. Eileen Ford (the founder of Ford Models, the internationally renowned modeling agency) used to tell me that she could always tell who was drinking enough water and who wasn't by the clarity and texture of their skin. That made a huge impression on me. Dehydration makes your skin less firm and elastic. You can't be Fit, Fab, and Fierce if you look run-down and dehydrated!

So, to recap, water:

- Acts like an appetite suppressant.
- Boosts your metabolism.
- Brightens your eyes and clears up your skin.
- Combats water retention.
- Improves your energy.
- Keeps you from getting dehydrated and eating when you're really thirsty.

I love fresh, plain water. But if you find it boring, sparkling water (plain or flavored with natural, calorie-free flavors) and mineral water add a little pizzazz and are also fine. Or, borrow a trick from high-class spas and infuse your water with fruits, vegetables, and/or spices and herbs to give it a little zing. Our Sugar Savvy Sisters LOVED their Spa Water, let me tell you. And because they loved it, they drank much, much more water than they ever have in their life!

There's no real magic to mixing Spa Water. Simply add a few slices or chunks of what you like to a pitcher of water and let it stand for a few hours before drinking. Refrigerate it if you like it chilled. Here are a few variations to try.

SPA WATER VARIATIONS

Cucumber Delite: Add slices of fresh cucumber.

Citrus Zing: Add sliced lemons, limes, and tangerines.

Ginger Goodness: Add some sliced fresh ginger.

Minty Fresh: Throw in some mint and rosemary sprigs.

Sweet Lavender: Just add fresh lavender sprigs and sliced strawberries.

Summer Melon: Add chunks of watermelon and mint sprigs.

You're really limited only by your imagination! Spa Water is pretty to look at, refreshing to drink, and good for you. So chugalug!

Coffee, Tea, and Me?

Can you drink coffee? Yes. Can you drink tea? Yes. Can you drink a Venti Frappuccino with extra whipped cream? Not a good idea! You may have your coffee and tea without sugar and with a bit of milk. I use just enough milk to cool off my coffee.

(continued on page 100)

Yoselis Balbi, Age 38
Aris Pacheco, Age 35

They both **learned the joy of cooking!**

Together lost 28 lbs and 15¼ inches in 6 weeks!

Friends Yoselis and Aris watched in amazement as their mutual pal Madeline De La Cruz (one of Voltage's Energy Up! girls) dropped more than 50 pounds and became 100 percent Fit, Fabulous, and Fierce. After years of battling their own weight, they wanted in!

"I've always struggled with my weight, despite being on dozens of diets," says Yoselis. "Once I start eating, I can't stop, especially carbs and bread. I was tired all the time. I wanted a complete lifestyle change."

"I was always a skip-dinner-and-go-straight-for-dessert kind of woman," says Aris. "I gained weight after my kids were born. I joined a gym and went on one diet after another. Nothing ever worked. My kids are 13 and 16. It's been too long. I need a change!"

Aris and Yoselis joined forces to become Sugar Savvy Sisters. They bought food scales, hit the stores,

> "We really enjoyed shopping, cooking, and learning to be Sugar Savvy together."

read labels, and learned how to make Sugar Savvy meals. "I was pretty nervous," confided Yoselis. "I kept thinking, 'I don't know if I'm going to be able to do this. I don't cook!' Well, I'm amazed! It's so easy that even I can do it! I can make a meal in 15 minutes that tastes really good!"

The sugar shockers helped scare both of them into trying healthier foods. "Once I learned how much sugar was in all those things I was eating, I didn't want them anymore! I don't even look at cookies and cakes. I don't crave them," says Aris.

"I've also discovered so many foods I never, ever would have tried, like Kamut, which is awesome," says Yoselis, who lost 15.4 pounds and 5¼ inches during the 6-week plan. "I eat it instead of pasta. It took me about a week to get the hang of the formulas, but it was so, so worth it. I never would have imagined I could lose all this weight. My knees don't hurt anymore. Before, I would be like, 'Wait. I have to stop and rest.' Now I can walk fast and keep up with everybody. I feel like I can do anything now."

"The best part is that I am in control," concluded Aris, who lost 12.6 pounds and 10 inches during the 6-week plan. "Nobody is going to tell me what I can and can't eat. I'm not afraid to make special orders at restaurants or friends' houses. I don't come home and go right to sleep anymore! I go to the gym. I cook dinner. I have so much more energy! I love being in control of my life."

> **Yoselis's and Aris's favorite affirmation:**
> I am happy! I am healthy! I am the best!
> And I deserve the best!

Sugar Savvy Hydration Trick

Having trouble remembering to drink, drink, drink? Try this Sugar Savvy trick: Each morning, place eight bracelets (bangles, bands, beads, whatever you like!) on your left wrist. Every time you drink 8 ounces of water, move the bracelet to the right. If you have any bracelets remaining on your left arm at the end of the day, you're not hydrating enough. Works like a charm!!

(continued from page 97)

Though coffee and tea are not the terrible diuretics they were once believed to be, they're still not great for hydration and on the Sugar Savvy program, they DO NOT count towards your quota of 64 ounces of water a day. Only water or sparkling water or mineral water (see the trend here?) count toward that!

Also, while you're making these positive changes, why not make one more and cut back on the java for a few weeks and see how you feel? I'll bet that once you're properly hydrated and not completely sapped by sugar, you'll be sparkling with so much energy that you won't be hunting for a Starbucks fix every hour. You'll also be calmer, feel less jittery, and sleep better. Plus you'll have more cash in your pocket from not plunking down 10 bucks a day on coffee drinks! I'm actually saving you money!

You Booze, You Lose (but Not Weight!)

I'm guessing you figured this out, but I'll spell it out for you just in case. Alcohol is NOT compatible with the Sugar Savvy solution, especially when your goal is to lose weight. I don't drink because I'm an alcoholic. Alcohol does not work for me. You might not be addicted to alcohol in the same way you're addicted to sugar, but it still interferes with the weight-loss and empowerment process. The calories and sugar in alcohol count as much as the calories and sugar in food. Alcohol also sharpens your appetite and clouds your judgement, which can lead to overeating. Even Sugar Savvy Sisters who wouldn't otherwise dream of touching fried food lose their resolve to resist wings, nachos, and French fries after a couple of drinks.

If you want to experience the full power of the Sugar Savvy solution, no drinking is a no-exception rule. In the end, some Sugar Savvy Sisters do choose to take a drink every now and then because their weight is stable, they eat very cleanly otherwise, and they can have one drink without it turning into three or four—or the whole bottle! After you reach your goals, your alcohol use is your personal choice, but for the 6 weeks of the Sugar Savvy program, please do abstain. Once you experience the natural high you get from being Sugar Savvy, you might not miss the buzz you get from drinking!

FOLLOW THE SUGAR SAVVY MEAL PLAN

If most of your food came in boxes and plastic bags up until this point, you can fully expect that much of the Sugar Savvy Meal Plan will look like Greek to you! But rest assured, it will soon be second nature! The Sugar Savvy solution is indeed a process, like learning a new language. And it *does* take time. The words are different. The structure is different. But once you get the basics down, you'll be able to carry on a fluent, beautiful conversation! Do not be hard on yourself during this process! What you're taking on is HUGE. But very doable! Keep the faith!

Each and every one of our successful Sugar Savvy Sisters said the same thing: ***It's hard in the beginning, but it just gets easier and easier!*** "There were all these foods, like tahini, that I didn't know what they were and it was taking me forever to make my meals because it was all so unfamiliar," says Lisa Brooks, 49. "But by Week 2, I got the hang of it and got into a rhythm. Now it's a breeze."

Even those who NEVER cooked were amazed at how quickly they became accomplished Sugar Savvy "chefs"! "I was very worried at the beginning of this plan because there were all these meals to make and I don't cook. But I decided to try," recalls Yoselis Balbi. "I bought a food scale and went shopping and followed the meal plan formulas and was shocked. The meals are so easy to make! In 15 minutes I can make food for 3 days! And the food tastes good! I really didn't think it was possible!"

Honestly, I was in the exact same boat! Though I've always eaten very Sugar Savvy, I confess that I bought a lot of my food instead of cooking myself. But once Jessica showed me how easy it was, I was really excited to see all the delicious meals I could make! Believe me. If *I* can do it, anyone can!

On the Sugar Savvy Meal Plan, you'll enjoy four Power Meals and one Power Drink per day. These mini-meals are all full of natural Sugar Savvy foods designed to provide you with MAXIMUM NUTRITION so you feel ALIVE with ENERGY. If you're allergic to or just don't like one of the meals or drinks in this sample week, no problem! In Chapter 10, I'll show you just how easy it is to create your own Power Meals using simple formulas plus a full list of delicious Sugar Savvy approved foods, while in Chapter 11, you'll find 40 Power Meals and Drinks you can mix and match as you like. To get started today, try this Sugar Savvy sample menu for a busy workweek. See Appendix A (page 242) for a shopping list to make it even easier to hit the ground running.

Day 1

Power Meal 1: Eggs over Greens and Grains (page 194)
Power Drink: Almond-Orange-Pineapple (page 215)
Power Meal 2: Broccoli and Chickpea Salad (page 199)
Power Meal 3: Open-Faced Tuna Salad Sandwich (page 202)
Power Meal 4: Warm Vegetable Medley (page 201)

Day 2

Power Meal 1: Oatmeal with Almonds and Blueberries (page 192)
Power Drink: Cucumber-Grape (page 214)
Power Meal 2: "Grilled" Veggie Salad (page 198)
Power Meal 3: Avocado and Cottage Cheese Dippers (page 200)
Power Meal 4: Veggie Stir-Fry (page 212)

Day 3

Power Meal 1: Avocado Egg Scramble (page 193)
Power Drink: Almond-Orange-Pineapple (page 215)
Power Meal 2: Broccoli and Chickpea Salad (page 199)
Power Meal 3: Open-Faced Tuna Salad Sandwich (page 202)
Power Meal 4: Beans 'n' Greens Pasta (page 209)

Day 4

Power Meal 1: Oatmeal with Almonds and Blueberries (page 192)
Power Drink: Cucumber-Grape (page 214)
Power Meal 2: "Grilled" Veggie Salad (page 198)
Power Meal 3: Roasted Eggplant and Tomato Sandwich (page 206)
Power Meal 4: Barley, Artichoke, and Chicken Salad (page 195)

Day 5

Power Meal 1: Cottage Cheese Medley (page 191)
Power Drink: Spinach-Orange-Banana (page 214)
Power Meal 2: Veggie Chili (page 207)
Power Meal 3: Avocado and Cottage Cheese Dippers (page 200)
Power Meal 4: Simple Salmon Salad (page 198)

MOVE YOUR BODY!

Remember how smoking used to be "normal"? Well, today there's a daily pastime that is every bit as normal and every bit as bad for you—sitting! Surveys show that the average woman and man now spend more than 56 hours a week—8 full hours a day—planted on their behinds like a potted fern! We sit in our cars. We sit at our desks. We sit in front of the TV at night. We sit in front of our computers. We use the Internet to shop, bank,

Stick-to-It Tricks

"It's hard work to eat right," Nancy told me on the phone one evening. "I can't just run out and grab something on the go. I have to plan this out."

Then there was this message from Catherine after our first meeting: "All right. It took me almost 5 hours, including shopping, chopping, cooking, and emulsifying, to make Soupalicious. The good news is, it made up a ton and the even better news is it tastes amazing. It was worth it but I am 'soup-er' tired so I am going to bed. . . . Phew!"

Damn right, it's work. I'm not one to sugarcoat (pun intended!) the facts. Getting Sugar Savvy is a big, life-altering change. LIFE-ALTERING CHANGES ARE NEVER EASY. They require EDUCATION and PREPARATION and PRACTICE! Remember, it's just the transition that is hard—it's not hard forever!

Consider the time you're putting in now an investment in your future. Right now, everything feels like so much work because you have to THINK so much! Before, you'd automatically (and mindlessly) wander to the vending machine for a pack of M&Ms. You'd nuke frozen dinners full of ingredients you didn't even understand. Sure, it was easy, but look where it got you!

Remember your affirmations. Remember what you want from your life! Repeat it. Repeat it. Repeat it. The more trips you make to the grocery store and the more Sugar Savvy meals you make, the more automatic and easy this way of life will become.

and even socialize without ever leaving our chair! And it's killing us!

You'll be starting the full Sugar Savvy Power Workout next week. But in the meantime, starting this week, I want you to **move your body for a minimum of 30 minutes a day**— walk, dance, run, hula hoop—whatever motivates you. Fit, Fab, and Fierce bodies were designed to move! Long before there was a "fitness industry" to follow, I've been preaching it, getting girls and women off their seats and on their feet, jumping and dancing and moving their muscles for 30 years. It was fun and exciting and I always knew deep in my heart that it was what our bodies and our minds needed! Now science has once again caught up to me and is showing that moving your body all day every day is far more important than anyone— even the exercise scientists—ever imagined!

Your body is a lot like the computer many of us spend so much time in front of. So long as we keep it active, it keeps whirring and running. What happens when you let it sit too long without use? *It goes to SLEEP!* The screen goes blank and it POWERS DOWN. That is EXACTLY what happens to your body when you sit,

sit, sit! Your body goes into conservation mode and starts SHUTTING DOWN!

You have special proteins and enzymes whose job it is to absorb fat and sugar out of the bloodstream. Well, those enzymes literally shut off and stop working when you sit for several hours without interruption. That means, the more you sit, the more fat and blood that remain in circulation, leaving you susceptible to all kinds of health problems.

Nonstop sitting is so bad for you that doctors now call it "sitting disease," and the consequences are grim. Every 2 hours you spend sitting at the job without taking a break to stand increases the likelihood you'll end up with type 2 diabetes by 7 percent. Spending all day parked on your butt also jacks up your risk for heart disease, depression, back pain, and even cancer. Most startling, researchers who examined the health and lifestyle habits of tens of thousands of people recently discovered that the more you sit each day, the more likely you are to die an early death *no matter how fit you are*. It's THAT important to move!

I realize that many working people today are forced to be at their desks for hours and hours at a time, but that doesn't mean you have to sit! Create a new normal working environment where you stand up and stretch every 30 minutes and stand for longer whenever possible. You can make your calls standing up. Sort through your in-box standing up. If you have a smartphone, you can even answer emails while standing and pacing.

Speaking of smartphones, I also recommend using this amazing technology to help you make the move to the new normal of Sugar Savvy living. If your smartphone has a built-in GPS, you can download apps like Moves and Garmin Fit that track your activity levels and Nike Training Club, which puts dozens of stretches and other easy, do-anywhere exercises right at your fingertips. Set reminders on your laptop and phone to stand up at regular intervals. Before long, standing and moving around will simply be "normal" behavior—what you do because it's what you want to do!

CHAPTER 6

WEEK 3: POWER UP WITH THE SUGAR SAVVY WORKOUT

Kick things up a notch with the Moving Affirmations and Power Workout; calm your cravings with the recharging station.

"I've always been very active but the Sugar Savvy Workout takes physical activity to another level by adding in the positive affirmations. It's fun and energizing and empowering."

—CATHERINE SCHULLER, 58, WHO LOST **11.2 POUNDS** IN **6 WEEKS**

Sugar Savvy Foundations

This week, as we build, continue to:

* Read your labels: Keep sugar sleuthing!

* Say and write your daily affirmations!

* Eat no more than 24 grams of added sugar in 24 hours.

* Hydrate right (drink eight 8-ounce glasses of water a day).

* Follow the Sugar Savvy Meal Plan.

* Move your body at least 30 minutes a day.

Sugar Savvy eating is absolutely essential. Keep following the Sugar Savvy Meal Plan this week, and don't forget to hydrate right! But all the healthy food in the world will only do you so much good if you spend your days parked on your behind! We keep the momentum rolling this week with the amazing Sugar Savvy Moving Affirmations and Power Workout. I will also introduce my secret weapon for staying centered and energized through even the most challenging of days—the Sugar Savvy recharging station!

THE SUGAR SAVVY MOVING AFFIRMATIONS

Do you find exercise boring? Me, too! That's why I created the Sugar Savvy Moving Affirmations. Because they are NOT your typical rote exercise routine. They are not just another ho-hum treadmill walk. The Moving Affirmations reprogram your *mind*—how you think about yourself and your life—while you give your body the movement it needs and craves. They energize your body, mind, and spirit. I do these with my Energy Up! students and *it literally changes their lives!* The more they perform them, the better they feel, the more they really believe in their own power to change.

When the nightclub at the spa I directed got a new sound system, I put the old one in the gym, making the health club a dance club. That's where I created these routines. On the dance floor, I felt a natural high I had never felt before, which was a *huge* revelation for me. I had feared I'd never feel high or happy again after getting sober! But when I did these routines, I'd reach this amazing state of euphoria and start *whoo*-ing! *Whoo!* is my personal Energy Up! motto. When I want a quick lift, I let out a *whoo!* It works every time! I answer the phone with a *whoo!* I say hello with a *whoo!* I knew our Sugar Savvy Sisters were on their way to a complete transformation when they started *whoo*-ing! *Whoo*-ing is my thing.

You've already learned how powerful affirmations can be. Now we're going to crank them up another notch. With the Moving Affirmations, you'll take some of my most powerful positive affirmations and set them to music and movement. Shout the affirmations and let out your *whoos* to wake up and fully engage your mind and your muscles. You may feel self-conscious or sluggish when you start, but I guarantee you'll be buzzing and raring to go 5 minutes in. When you say things out loud and proud with power and strength, you believe them and make them true. That's what the Moving Affirmations are all about.

> Think of the Moving Affirmations as **boot camp** not just for your muscles, but also your mind!

The magic happens by blending the movement and the words. Because as you reach that endorphin-fueled state, your brain will be open and ready to soak in and accept your affirmations as reality. It's amazingly powerful! You'll find the complete description of the Moving Affirmations in Chapter 12 on pages 220–225. Remember that it's essential that you harness your powerful spirit when you do them and bring it out in full force. That you BELIEVE that you **can** do this. That you BELIEVE that you can do anything! Think of it as boot camp for not just for your muscles, but also your mind! Ideally, you should do the entire 30-minute series every day. But **I want you to do at least two Moving Affirmations each day.** These can be done on their own (maybe in the morning, when you first get up). Or they make the perfect warm-up for the Sugar Savvy Power Workout. That's how we did them with the Sugar Savvy Sisters, and by the time we hit the weights, those women were REVVED UP and ready to rock!

(continued on page 112)

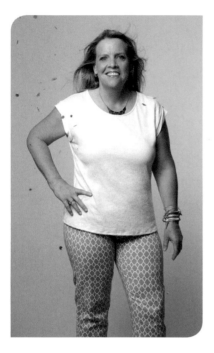

Nancy Barthold, Age 51

Nancy **shot up a whopping 12 points** on the Rosenberg Self-Esteem Scale as she learned to manage her food addiction.

Lost 11.2 lbs and 8¾ inches in 6 weeks!

Like Voltage (and millions of others), Nancy is a classic food addict. Once she starts eating her trigger foods, she simply can't stop. She doesn't eat when she's hungry. She eats whenever she can, all day every day, whether it's muffins in a work meeting or—her binge of choice—a bag of popcorn and a carton of ice cream at night. She came to the Sugar Savvy plan because it wasn't just another diet—it was a ticket to freedom from food addiction.

"I'm extremely active. I do triathlons. But you would never know it to look at me. I want to look as active as I am," she says. "I also want to be healthy. My mother had a massive stroke when she was 65 and then went on to develop diabetes. She died of cardiac arrest 10 years ago. I asked my doctor how I could avoid the same fate and he told me that I needed to get control of my out-of-control eating."

> ## "I was finally able to face down my food addiction."

Nancy used the Palate Cleanse as a chance to hit "reboot" on her eating habits. She also zoned in on the Sugar Savvy star point of having an attitude of gratitude. "After a few days of the cleanse, I really didn't crave popcorn and ice cream. And I'm more mindful now. I get up and write what I'm going to eat for the day. Instead of just grabbing and stuffing food in my mouth, I sit down, pause, center myself, and recognize that I am eating. I acknowledge that this is one of several meals I will have today and I should appreciate it. That extra acknowledgment helps me recognize that food is fuel rather than just enter-tainment. I finally know what real hunger feels like, and I like it," she says.

Because Nancy lives in a big city, where there's food at every turn, she knows now that she must always be prepared! "That's the hardest part. I need to get better about preparing my food so I always have it on me," she says. "I'm active. I ride my bike and I train. So I need to be prepared to add a Sugar Savvy meal or snack like sprouted bread with almond butter when I know I'll be on a long ride. It is a little harder to be spontaneous, but it's really worth it. It's a lifestyle that makes sense. I love feeling the benefits. My jeans have been tight. They are now loose. I'm getting there, one day at a time."

Nancy's favorite affirmation: I am happy! I am healthy! I am beautiful and strong!

(continued from page 109)

Note: If you already have a regular workout routine, you can do the series as a warm-up; perform it on days you're not doing other exercise, or simply pick your favorite two or three exercises to do daily for an added boost!

> Lean muscle raises your metabolism, helps manage blood sugar levels, and looks **Fit, Fab, and Fierce!**

THE SUGAR SAVVY POWER WORKOUT

This week it's also time to start making some muscle! As I mentioned earlier, lean muscle tissue raises your metabolism (which means faster weight loss) and helps pull glucose (i.e., SUGAR) from your bloodstream to manage your blood sugar levels. Plus, let's face it, toned muscles look Fit, Fab, and Fierce! The moves in the Sugar Savvy Power Workout tap into all your major muscles and will help make you stronger and more energetic for everything you do!

If you've tried any strength-training plans before, you've probably heard that you need to rest for a day in between workouts to recover. While the Power Workout does work your muscles, it's designed to be a bit more gentle than hard-core bodybuilding routines. This simple routine takes about 30 minutes and sculpts, strengthens, and stretches your body, so it's very efficient! You can do it as often as you feel moved to—I do it every day—but **aim for at least 3 or 4 days a week.** If you already strength-train on your own, by all means keep at it! Or give this workout a try for some variety. You'll find the full Sugar Savvy Power Workout in Chapter 12 on pages 228–231.

I would also like you to stretch every day. There's some stretching built into the Power Workout already, but you can never do too much—***stretching is so important for your body and soul!*** The best part is you can do it no matter where you are! A good stretch not only helps keep you flexible, it also provides a quick hit of energy! Throughout the day I will stretch my arms out to the sides and then stretch them over my head while inhaling deeply through my nose, then let my breath out through my mouth, thinking *positive ENERGY in . . . negative ENERGY out!!!!* So be sure to take plenty of stretch breaks throughout the day every day!

THE RECHARGING STATION

Like most of us, your life is filled with demands and must-dos! Many, many energy sappers out there can bring even the strongest Sugar Savvy Sister down! To be successful on this journey, you need to be able to recharge your batteries on a regular basis.

This week I want you to **create your own recharging station.** Find a corner in your room and/or at work if that's a place of high stress for you. Decorate it with an object that reinforces your new commitment to live the Sugar Savvy life. It can be an aromatherapy candle, a colorful light, a special talisman, or a personal memento that empowers you. Maybe it's just a written list of your favorite affirmations. Here's one I really like for recharging:

> ✳ I am happy, I am healthy!
> And I choose to be powerful, strong, filled with energy!

Go there at least once a day. Say your affirmations and take a few minutes to remember why you started this journey, and steel your resolve to be Fit, Fabulous, and Fierce!

It really doesn't take much. Sugar Savvy Sister Cheryl Lee used a simple vase of fresh-cut flowers as a reminder of all the beauty—and the power of beauty—in this world! Nancy Barthold took it one step further by finding a place by the Hudson River outside her office to go to for 15 minutes a day to clear her head, center herself, and recharge before returning to her high-stress job.

CHAPTER 7

WEEK 4: KICK SUGAR'S EVIL SIDEKICKS TO THE CURB

Dig deeper to eliminate all triggers while you sidestep excess salt, nasty fat, and enriched white flour.

"Some people can eat whole grain breads and pastas. I can't. Those are just trigger foods for me. I'm a carb lover—too much so! I need to keep it to fruits and veggies and sweet potatoes, or I go overboard and gain weight. Through this program I've been able to see the direct effect of my actions. When I stay away from those trigger foods—even though they're healthy—I lose weight. When I don't, I don't lose weight. Usually I even gain some."

—CHERYL LEE, 50, WHO LOST **18.6 POUNDS** IN **6 WEEKS**

Sugar Savvy Foundations

This week, as we build, continue to:

* Read your labels: Keep sugar sleuthing!

* Say and write your daily affirmations!

* Eat no more than 24 grams of added sugar in 24 hours.

* Hydrate right (drink eight 8-ounce glasses of water a day).

* Follow the Sugar Savvy Meal Plan.

* Practice your Moving Affirmations and Power Workout.

* Visit your recharging station daily.

By now you should be getting the hang of the Sugar Savvy Meal Plan. Hopefully you've discovered some new favorite foods, including the Power Meals and Drinks you can always count on to satisfy you. But the novelty and excitement of starting a new plan may be wearing off, so maybe your weight loss has stalled or you've even regained a pound or two. Don't lose faith! Keep up your Moving Affirmations and the Power Workout, and get ready to dig deeper. Don't forget to keep visiting your recharging station and writing down your affirmations morning and night; you'll really need that reinforcement as you tackle your emotional triggers.

ELIMINATE ALL TRIGGERS

Now is the time to really dig in and fully commit. This week I want you to pull each and every trigger food from your diet. Get them out of your kitchen. Get them out of the snack drawer in your office. Get them out of your life!

Go back to the Trigger Food Trap Quiz (page 53) and identify ALL your triggers. You might find that even some Sugar Savvy–approved foods can be triggers for you. Supercharged Carbs, for instance, proved to be problematic for several Sugar Savvy Sisters, such as Cheryl. For some people (like me!), even healthy grains and whole grain–based foods like brown rice can trigger a binge.

If this is true for you, **cut grains, bread, crackers, and pasta out completely** this week. We'll talk about adding them back at a later time. But it is important to get them out this week to see how you feel. You need to see how awesome and in control and energized you CAN feel when you're not walking around like a mindless eating machine all day, which is how trigger foods—***even if they are otherwise healthy***—can make you act and feel! When you eat a trigger food, there simply is no off switch—this is not emotional, it's physical.

Inevitably when I talk about pulling out all these foods, someone will ask, "When can I eat grains [or even worse, cookies and cakes] again?" That question is simply not in our conversation right now! First you MUST find out what works for you. THEN you can figure out how to eat whatever it is that you want in a healthy, responsible way! Just as we need to learn to drink responsibly, we need to learn to eat responsibly.

Remember, the destination of this journey is to **eat whatever you want**, as you will have ***changed*** what you want. You will learn to love REAL whole foods and will be able to enjoy your sweet tooth in a very HEALTHY, empowering way! I promise you at the end of this journey, if you want a cookie, you can have a cookie. It might be a different kind of cookie than the ones that used to "set you off." For instance, I have found a vegan bakery that makes cupcakes and other sweets that are not as sugary and refined, so I can have just one without losing control (although I never bring them home). But I don't recommend experimenting with sweets until you're firmly on the Sugar Savvy track. Right now, I need you to stay focused on what will bring you to your goal and to being a true Sugar Savvy Sister who is Fit, Fab, and Fierce in every way. And right now that means we don't like cookies!

Also this week, **revisit your trigger emotions and situations**. Have you made progress in those areas of your life that leave you stressed, sad, and looking for a food fix? (And are you carrying your Sugar Savvy foods with you, so you'll have them when you need one?) Commit to changing those areas in your life that you can control.

TAKE A SECOND LOOK AT THOSE LABELS

By this point, you've likely gotten the sugar sleuthing down and are vigilant about consuming no more than 24 grams of added sugar in 24 hours. But remember, sugar isn't the only unhealthy ingredient food manufacturers use to get you hooked on junk food! As I talked about in Chapter 2, they also use ample amounts of sugar's evil sidekicks: excess salt, nasty fat, and enriched white flour. Even if you get rid of all the added sugar in your diet, you could still be stuck with 4 to 6 pounds of bloat because of all the extra salt in your diet. And you can't be Fit, Fab, and Fierce if you're weighed down with flour—just think of the silhouette of the Pillsbury Doughboy!

Four weeks into the plan, Jackie Georgantzas thought she and her mom Arlene were doing everything right. They were following the Power Meal formulas as best they could and watching their added sugar intake. But Jackie was getting a bit frustrated. Her weight seemed stuck. You guessed it—it was those evil sidekicks. Jackie saw firsthand how hidden sodium can put on pounds fast.

"We found that we needed to go out to eat less and cook our own food more often," said Jackie. "Even when I thought I was being healthy and ordering the vegetable soup or the bean soup, it would be loaded with salt. Now we go out once or twice a week and eat at home the rest of the time. That way we can really control what we're eating. I'm excited to see how quickly you make progress when you focus on doing it right. I've never been this serious about something before, but I can see how my cravings really do go away and I feel so much better when I do it right."

By following the Sugar Savvy Meal Plan, you should already be mostly free from excess salt, nasty fat, and enriched white flour. But as Jackie's example shows, if you're still eating out, buying take-out, and/or buying packaged foods, you may be consuming more salt, fat, and flour (and maybe even sugar) than you think.

That's why this week I'd like you to **examine all your food labels and ingredients** to make sure excess salt, fat, and flour haven't snuck in to sabotage your Sugar Savvy efforts. Remember, this exercise isn't intended to drive you crazy counting fat grams or calculating sodium amounts; I just want you to become aware of how much salt, unhealthy fat, and enriched white flour are present in packaged and processed foods (even healthy-sounding ones like the whole grain bread whose nutrition label is depicted below) so you can remove them and make room for all your new Sugar Savvy solution foods!

When buying packaged foods, here's what you're looking for:

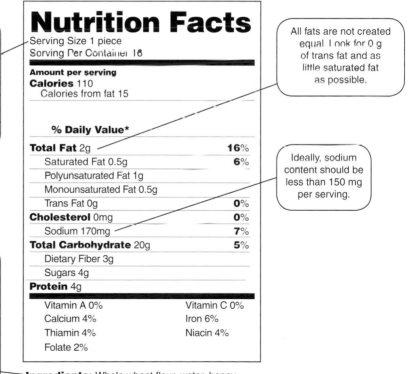

Look at serving sizes and the total number of servings. This example is for a loaf of bread. Note that the serving size is 1 piece but most people eat 2 slices at a time (if they're making sandwiches).

Nutrition Facts
Serving Size 1 piece
Serving Per Container 18

Amount per serving
Calories 110
    Calories from fat 15

% Daily Value*

Total Fat 2g	**16**%
Saturated Fat 0.5g	**6**%
Polyunsaturated Fat 1g	
Monounsaturated Fat 0.5g	
Trans Fat 0g	**0**%
Cholesterol 0mg	**0**%
Sodium 170mg	**7**%
Total Carbohydrate 20g	**5**%
Dietary Fiber 3g	
Sugars 4g	
Protein 4g	

Vitamin A 0%	Vitamin C 0%
Calcium 4%	Iron 6%
Thiamin 4%	Niacin 4%
Folate 2%	

All fats are not created equal. Look for 0 g of trans fat and as little saturated fat as possible.

Ideally, sodium content should be less than 150 mg per serving.

Make sure sugar (or a version of sugar), salt, and enriched white flour are NOT one of the first three ingredients. And look for how many types of sugar there are. In this example, there are three: honey (one of the first three ingredients), sugar, and unsulphured molasses.

Ingredients: Whole wheat flour, water, honey, yeast, wheat gluten, soy fiber, soybean oil. Contains 2 percent or less of: unsulphured molasses, nonfat milk, salt, butter, datem, vegetable mono and diglycerides, calcium propionate, soy lecithin and enzymes.

(continued on page 122)

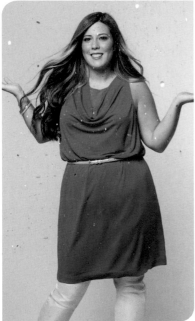

Cassandra Silva, Age 21

She **doesn't have headaches** nearly every day anymore. She doesn't have them at all!

Lost 10.8 lbs and 6¾ inches in 6 weeks!

When it comes to weight loss, Cassandra has always had an all-or-nothing attitude. "I would eat fast food all day, even for breakfast. I would start each day with a big bacon, egg, and cheese sandwich," she says. "Until I wanted to lose weight. Then I would try just eating salads until I never wanted to eat a salad again. I'd get so hungry and miserable, I'd go back to McDonald's." But she was so tired of being overweight and feeling lousy, she knew she had to find a sustainable solution.

Admittedly, she was skeptical at first about the Sugar Savvy solution. "I wasn't sure about this when I started," she says. "I figured it'd be another diet that would leave me miserable and feeling deprived. But once I saw how much sugar was in everything and how bad it was not just for my weight but my body, I really didn't want it. I wanted better for myself."

She took the Sugar Savvy Meal Plan home and, with the help of her mother, started cooking healthy meals that actually left her satisfied. "We've been

> ## "I don't miss fast food—at all!"

making brown rice and beans and a larger variety of healthy foods, so it's not like I'm just eating salads," she says. "In the morning I have Greek yogurt and muesli. I feel healthy. I used to have headaches all the time. I haven't had headaches. I haven't had any fast food. I don't want it."

Even better, both her parents followed in her footsteps. "They were both diagnosed with very high blood pressure, so they decided to try the program, too, since it's low in salt as well as sugar. Now whenever we go out, we can't stand the taste of most restaurant food. It's SO salty!" she says.

The change has been working for all of them. Her parents' blood pressure is coming down and Cassandra's weight is coming off. After 15 weeks of eating Sugar Savvy, she was down 23.5 pounds and still losing! "The steady weight loss is very motivating to help me stick with it," she says. "I've changed what I want. I have to admit, I miss bacon. I work at a deli where there's lots of bacon always cooking and yes, I still want it. But the few times I've eaten the bacon, or other fried foods, I've gotten a stomachache. My whole body has CHANGED what it wants! Maybe over time I'll completely lose my craving for it. All I know is I'm sticking with this lifestyle because it works!"

> **Cassandra's favorite affirmation: I am happy! I am healthy! I am powerful and strong!**

(continued from page 119)

HANDLE SLIP-UPS WITH POSITIVE AFFIRMATIONS

Are you still writing down your affirmations? I hope so! Now is also the time to make some new ones! When you say something over and over to yourself, your subconscious mind accepts it as truth! That's why it's VERY important that when any of those tired negative voices comes creeping back, you STOP it in its tracks and replace it with one of your positive affirmations, pronto!

> When you say something over and over to yourself, your subconscious mind **accepts it as truth!**

This is especially important during this phase of the Sugar Savvy plan, when there will be times when you "blow it" by forgetting you don't like or need CRAP food anymore and eat a bag of chips or a few brownies at a party and are tempted to lay into yourself. Don't! Instead, hold your head high and say, "I just forgot that I don't want those foods anymore. I remember now," and repeat your affirmations. It will quickly empower you to get right back on track!

One trick that Cheryl used was to use a different positive affirmation every day, which I fully support because it really makes you THINK about who you want to be and how you want to view yourself in that particular moment, under whatever circumstances you face right then! She has a beautiful routine that she performs each morning to get her into the Sugar Savvy mind-set.

"I pray and then I look at myself in the mirror and say my affirmations. Then I have two glasses of water instead of what used to be my coffee and a cigarette," says Cheryl. "It's been a process, but it works. You can really change how you think, which changes your whole life. I have overcome being addicted to salty foods. I have overcome being addicted to carbs. I have overcome my dependence on processed foods. I have overcome insecure. I never thought I could do any of that. I am so grateful for i

I encouraged all the Sugar Savvy Sisters who tested this plan to make their own affirmations. I most certainly encourage you to make your own affirmations. But over the years I've seen that sometimes women are so used to thinking negative thoughts that they actually have a hard time coming up with positive ones! I gave you a few in Chapter 1 and even more in the Moving Affirmation series. But you're going to need more than that to be Sugar Savvy forever! So here is a list you can choose from, including some from our Sugar Savvy Sisters. Pick the ones that speak to you. Use them when you need them. And do try to come up with a few of your own!

* I am happy! I am healthy! There is nothing I can't do!

* I am happy! I am healthy! Nothing can bring me down!

* I am happy! I am healthy! I am a superstar!

* I am happy! I am healthy! I have a huge attitude filled with gratitude!

* I am happy! I am healthy! I am strong and powerful!

* I am happy! I am healthy! My heart is full of love!

* I am happy! I am healthy! Nothing can stop me!

* I am happy! I am healthy! My life is mine to own!

* I am happy! I am healthy! I can do anything!

* I am happy! I am healthy! It's a beautiful day in every way!

* I am happy! I am healthy! I am fearless and free!

* I am happy! I am healthy! I am full of pride! No reason to hide!

* I am happy! I am healthy! I'm sugar free and filled with energy!

CHAPTER 8

WEEK 5: GET STRESS SAVVY TO GET SUGAR SAVVY

Banish food addiction by taking charge of your attitude: Practice kindness, assume an attitude of gratitude and forgiveness, and choose happiness!

"I realized that I was lying to myself an awful lot. I would tell myself that my eating and drinking were making me happy when what I really needed to find happiness was to stop my unhealthy eating and drinking."

—PATRICIA NOLAN, 47, WHO LOST 15.8 POUNDS IN 6 WEEKS

Sugar Savvy Foundations

This week as we build, continue to:

* Read your labels: Keep sugar sleuthing!

* Say and write your daily affirmations!

* Eat no more than 24 grams of added sugar in 24 hours.

* Hydrate right (drink eight 8-ounce glasses of water a day).

* Follow the Sugar Savvy Meal Plan.

* Practice your Moving Affirmations and Power Workout

* Visit your recharging station daily.

* Kick your trigger foods to the curb.

* Push yourself to be Sugar Savvy 24/7.

As we move deeper into the 6-week Sugar Savvy plan, cooking up your meals and snacks should be becoming second nature. You should be shouting those affirmations loudly and proudly and moving your body throughout the day, every day. And you should be leaving old self-destructive behaviors behind as you adopt your Sugar Savvy attitude of gratitude! Keep recharging your batteries to stay on track. This week, we're going to concentrate on that attitude as we highlight the star points that focus on your emotional and mental health and empowerment—announcing your affirmations and assuming an attitude of gratitude and forgiveness.

CHOOSE JOY

You make dozens—maybe hundreds—of decisions every day that affect your happiness. Well, the very first decision you need to make is to **be happy!** Yes. That's right. Happiness is a CHOICE! Listen, life happens. On any given day we ALL have a lot of crap in our lives that we could use as an excuse to be unhappy, that we could wallow in, that we could use to justify burying ourselves in a box of cookies. ***Get over it.*** Make the choice EVERY DAY that you will be happy. The easiest way to snap out of your misery is to be grateful for what you have! Remember, there are women around the world who are property! They don't even own their own lives! You DO! Sitting around being miserable is a choice! Stop choosing it! Take control of your life. It's the only one you've got and ***you're*** the only one who can control how you respond to it!

Remember, too, that stress and unhappiness can make it harder to resist those so-called "comfort" foods that make you feel better for a split second before plunging you further into a funk! By choosing to be happy, you're already ahead of the game! The quizzes on pages 58 through 68 helped identify the areas in your life that may lead you to emotional eating. If you haven't already started, this week I want you to take action. Take steps to improve those areas of your life that are making you unhappy. Whether it's your job or your relationships or your jealous tendencies, NOW is the time to get on the path to improvement! You are not a victim of the food industry anymore, and you are not a victim of life!

> If you're someone who eats when they're stressed, you **must be prepared** to deal with that!

I *know* that sounds like an "easier said than done" charge. But it's NOT that complicated. Take ONE step, no matter how small, in the right direction. If your job makes you miserable, update your resume. If money woes are wearing you down, track your spending. If anger is eating you up, forgive. Every little step will lift you to a better place!

EAT TO BEAT STRESS

Because there's no way on earth you can fully avoid stress, I also want you to be prepared to respond to it. If you're someone who eats when they're stressed, you MUST BE PREPARED to deal with that! I can't tell you how many times I hear the same sad song about how "I can't help but eat when I'm stressed!" Well, I'm not going to tell you that you absolutely cannot eat when you're stressed. That'll just cause *more* stress! I'm telling you that you must be prepared with your Sugar Savvy foods within reach at all times so when you end up stressed and tired and hungry, you're not vulnerable to all the CRAP food that's tempting you at every turn! You are going to get stronger and stronger on this journey, and eventually you may even break that impulse to gorge just because you're stressed. However, the issue really isn't if you're eating or not eating, it's what you're eating! If you're bingeing on carrots and other veggies, it's not a problem!

The same goes for PMS. If it's that time of the month and all you want to do is eat, eat, eat, I'm not telling you not to eat, eat, eat. It's *what* you eat that matters! You need to **be prepared** and have your Sugar Savvy foods around you so you can make choices that will nourish and satisfy and energize you rather than turning you into a mindless, malnourished eating machine!

Sugar Savvy Stress-Beating Strategies

The Sugar Savvy plan is all about positive change. You are changing what you like, changing what you want, and changing the way you look at things. A large part of that is realizing that you cannot always change what happens in life, only how you feel about it and react to it. Over the course of the program, our Sugar Savvy Sisters developed many wonderful strategies for managing stress in a positive manner and preventing food cravings from taking over. Here are a few of my favorites.

* "As a pre-med student, I am often under a large amount of stress," says Madeline De La Cruz, 22, one of my original Energy Up! girls, who reached her goal weight following the Sugar Savvy program. "It's easy to be tempted by pastries and sweets when I'm studying and not exercising like I should be. But I try to use my daily affirmations to bring my thoughts back into positive focus. I even downloaded an app—Unique Daily Affirmations—that I can use for positive reinforcement. I find the urge for sweets passes when I stop and focus on being the best and doing the best for myself."

PRACTICE KARMIC KINDNESS AND ASSUME AN ATTITUDE OF GRATITUDE AND FORGIVENESS

Finally, this week I want you to be sure you're not just nourishing your mind and body, but also your soul. Starting right now, I want you **to perform at least one act of kindness every day**, and forgive someone, even yourself. So many of us get so wrapped up in me, me, me and what's going on in MY life that we forget about others. You are vitally important, of course. You have to love yourself first and foremost. But that love does no good unless you spread it around! Nurture that love for yourself and then share it with the world around you. The more you give, the more you have!

* "I personally live through a lot of stress," says Arlene Pineda, 58, who recently underwent surgery to have a pancreatic tumor removed. "But stressful situations make you grow emotionally and spiritually. I make an effort to stay connected with what is important. To that end, I've realized that I am important and I need to take care of myself—something that I am not always good at doing. I take care of my children, parents, family, and friends and place myself last. Even in my professional role, I take care of others first. By acknowledging myself as most important in my life, I stop and pause and make better decisions to care for myself, and this includes the way I eat."

* "When I have a bad day that would make the 'old me' binge, I ask myself what's really eating me before I start eating," says Catherine Schuller, 58. "I talk to myself in a kind and gentle, yet firm and strict way instead of just berating myself. It really works. Sometimes I still give in and take a little bite of what I want, but that's it, just a bite. Then I put it away. I haven't 'finished the bag' in a long, long, long time."

As part of the plan, I will ask that you to perform one act of kindness and express gratitude and forgiveness every day. What does being kind to other people have to do with losing weight and kicking food addiction?

Everything! Remember, many of us get hooked on sugar because it lights up all those feel-good reward centers in our brain. It makes us feel good when we're feeling bad.

> **Doing good feels good** and makes you less susceptible to seeking out sugar to lift your spirits.

Well, get this: ***Doing nice things for other people and forgiving them trips those same happy brain circuits!*** Neuroscientists at the National Institutes of Health did experiments scanning people's brains as they were told to imagine a scenario involving either donating money to a good cause or putting it in their own bank account. To their shock, they found that acting generously charged the same primitive parts of the brain that light up like a Christmas tree when we eat chocolate cake!

Doing good feels good and makes you less susceptible to backsliding into binge-eating and seeking out sugar to lift your spirits. When you forgive others or do something kind for them, you're truly also forgiving and doing something kind for yourself. Positive thinking and positive action make for very powerful medicine! Performing acts of kindness is about being humble, gentle, and caring to those around you. Those acts give you the power to cultivate a positive mental attitude so you don't waste your energy on negative thoughts and influences. When you see the light in someone's eyes when you're kind to them, it's the most awe-inspiring high of all.

What's more, doing good for others and contributing positively to those around you builds self-esteem. The higher your self-esteem, the less susceptible you are to self-destructive behaviors like binge-eating. It's also nearly impossible to feel negative emotional trigger feelings like loneliness and uselessness when you are out in the world helping other people!

So as part of the Sugar Savvy plan, you'll be expected and hopefully excited to perform one act of kindness and forgiveness daily, but you don't need to limit yourself! This is one place where I would encourage you to **binge with abandon!** Remember, this isn't about heroics. It's about looking up once in a while, noticing those around you, and saying or doing something sweet (not eating something sweet). These karmic acts of kindness can be especially powerful when you perform them in places typically rife with negative emotional triggers, like the workplace. A few simple examples:

- Compliment a stranger on her shoes/hairstyle/manicure.
- Thank a co-worker for her contributions to a project.
- Forgive your spouse for not noticing your new outfit.
- Open the door for someone whose hands are full.
- Surprise your sweetie with coffee in bed.
- Say a few kind words to someone you're jealous of.
- Perform one of the chores that's not typically yours (i.e., taking out the trash, even though your spouse or son usually does it).
- Let go of an old grudge and reach out to a friend you haven't talked to in a while.
- Drop off a bag of groceries at your local food bank.
- Volunteer at your child's or grandchild's school.
- Let someone go ahead of you in line at the bank, post office, or grocery store.
- Forgive the driver who cut you off.
- Give a family member an unexpected embrace.

(continued on page 134)

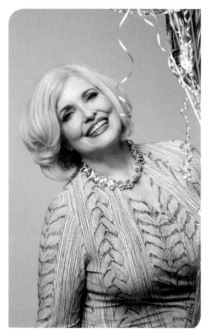

Catherine Schuller, Age 58

Catherine's triglyceride and blood pressure levels
dropped from high to normal.

As a plus-sized model, Catherine has always been comfortable in her curves. But over the years her weight crept up and her health declined. She came to the Sugar Savvy plan with prediabetes and metabolic syndrome, and three years into recovery from a stroke. She was already very active, riding her bike all over the city, and was a conscientious eater, avoiding obvious sugar and eating very little meat. She had lost about 40 pounds, but had 40 more to lose and was stuck. She was on multiple medications to lower her blood sugar, triglycerides, and blood pressure and her doctor wanted to prescribe more.

Lost 11.2 lbs and 4 inches in 6 weeks!

"I felt like he was pushing drugs on me and I wanted to fix this myself. I wanted to find the missing piece to getting healthy," she says. Turns out the biggest piece was portion control. "Though I was eating healthy foods, I was still always eating until I was stuffed. I've learned that I don't want to feel that way. I measure out my food and I pile on the veggies and I take my time to appreciate the food and when I'm done I tune in to myself and I've realized

> "I learned you can overeat good food, too. Now I'm working on getting my portions just right."

that I'm really okay. I'm not hungry. I'm satisfied. I haven't had that extra-full feeling since I've started this and I don't miss it," she says. "Now, if I make 2 or 3 servings of something, I'm sure to wrap up the extra for another meal. I also work hard to make my drinks and meals and even water as nutritious as possible."

Catherine also realized she was eating more sugar than she thought, because it was in places she didn't expect it, like "diet" foods. "This program has opened my mind to the Industrial Food Matrix. They can't have me. Even these so-called diet foods are completely processed, and many have added sugars and salts and chemicals. I refuse to be a sheep," she says. "We are waging the good fight. They can't get control over us; we are strong and powerful! Keep shopping and cooking and preparing—it will pay off!"

It surely has for Catherine! Her triglycerides dropped from 330 milligrams per deciliter to 64 (200–499 mg/dL is considered high; less than 150 is normal) and her blood pressure went from 165/90 millimeters of mercury to 123/79 (120/80 mmHg or lower is considered normal). So now she's off her triglyceride and blood pressure medications. "I hope to hit my goal weight in the next few weeks," she says. "This is a complete lifestyle change, but if you stay the course, I promise you'll be rewarded!"

Catherine's favorite affirmation: I am happy and healthy and even though I stray, I am still okay!

Take the Sugar Savvy Pledge!

Just as the students in my Energy Up! programs start their day with the Pledge of Allegiance to our country, I have them wrap up each session of our program with a pledge to themselves to live Sugar Savvy! This pledge is a powerful extension of the Sugar Savvy affirmations and a clear reminder of how to live a Fit, Fabulous, and Fierce life! Repeat after me!

I am HAPPY

I am HEALTHY

and I CHOOSE to be

Fit, Fab, Fierce and SUGAR SAVVY

I eat veggies and fruit EVERYDAY

PUSH salty foods out of the way

I move my body, JUMP, and SHOUT

Drink plenty of water

SUGAR IS OUT

I'm LOUD and PROUD

with a HUGE ATTITUDE

but it's cool you see it's

all GRATITUDE

(continued from page 131)

Like eating natural foods and moving your body, performing daily acts of kindness often becomes second nature when you do it enough! You'll crave the positive interaction with the world and miss it if you get too self-absorbed and caught up in those old, jealous, woe-is-me feelings for too long. You'll feel so good inside, you won't be searching for a sugar boost. As a bonus, you'll be making others feel better, too, so they'll be less inclined to binge to beat the blues. It's like dropping a **good-karma bomb** on the obesity crisis!

AMAZING GRACE

One of the ways I stay on track is spending time every single day being grateful for the amazing things in my life and how much better I feel. It's nearly impossible to give ANY power to a doughnut, when without one I have an energy level many 20-year-olds envy and am ready to rock and roll and enjoy a fantastic life!

Saying grace before meals is practically unheard of these days, but I believe it's a practice we should bring back no matter what our spiritual affiliation. Giving thanks for the nourishment on the table before you makes you want to put praiseworthy food on your plate! Would you be inclined to give thanks for a pile of Fritos and a Dr. Pepper? I don't think so! But you should be moved to give thanks for a bounty of fruits and vegetables and wonderful fish and poultry and other whole foods.

"I've really grown to appreciate the absolute beauty of Sugar Savvy foods," says Catherine. "I went to a friend's house and they had prepared the most gorgeous salad with all these brilliant colors and textures and it was so delicious. It's been a pleasure to discover how much more satisfying fresh, natural foods are on every level. We're so used to getting excited about cakes and desserts, but it's been a pleasure to discover how excited I've been about Sugar Savvy foods. Every time I go out to eat now I ask myself 'What is the healthiest thing I can order?' and I've found that many times I would return just for that dish!"

> Giving thanks for the nourishment on the table makes you want to put **praiseworthy food** on your plate!

Starting now, ***say a little prayer*** at the start of every meal. Even if you are just sitting down to a snack of carrots and hummus, take a moment, take a breath, and register the fact that you are about to eat. Appreciate your food. Be present. Then eat mindfully and with grace. At the end of each day, bring to mind at least three things you're grateful for.

CHAPTER 9

WEEK 6: SUGAR SAVVY FOR LIFE

Find your new normal and feel Fit, Fab, and Fierce!

"This is not a diet. This is not a fad. This is not something I'm just doing for a while. This is the new me. This is how I live now. There's no going back."

—ARIS PACHECO, 35, WHO LOST 12.6 POUNDS IN 6 WEEKS

Sugar Savvy Foundations

This week as we build, continue to:

* Read your labels: Keep sugar sleuthing!

* Say and write your daily affirmations!

* Eat no more than 24 grams of added sugar in 24 hours.

* Hydrate right (drink eight 8-ounce glasses of water a day).

* Follow the Sugar Savvy Meal Plan.

* Practice your Moving Affirmations and Power Workout

* Visit your recharging station daily.

* Kick your trigger foods to the curb.

* Push yourself to be Sugar Savvy 24/7.

* Adopt an attitude of gratitude and forgiveness and perform one kind act a day.

As you enter the sixth and final week of the Sugar Savvy solution, it's time to look back at what has worked for you thus far as well as ahead toward what you can maintain for life. What has changed about what you want? What are some of your newfound favorites? Remember, this is no temporary diet. You should still be living, eating, and moving according to the Sugar Savvy solution—making Sugar Savvy meals, performing your Moving Affirmations, adopting an attitude of gratitude and forgiveness each and every day! This is a high-wattage approach to fueling your body in a way that will help you stay Fit, Fabulous, and Fierce for life!

At this point you should find that you really no longer want dead, sugar-laden foods that sap your energy minutes after you've wiped the crumbs from your lips.

That said, it's natural to occasionally forget that you don't want certain foods any longer. Often, girls in the Energy Up! program come to me as though I'm a priest awaiting confession and come clean about some dietary indiscretion. "I have to tell you, Voltage," they'll begin, "I was at a party and everyone was eating chips and pizza. And I thought I would have some, too. But they weren't as good as I remembered them being. They were actually pretty gross."

That's exactly what Sugar Savvy is all about! It's not to say that you will never, ever have a piece of cake or potato chip again, but that they aren't as appealing to you as they used to be. You may occasionally forget that you don't like those old foods anymore and help yourself to a serving. But chances are, you'll soon discover they just aren't what you want anymore. You'll quickly remember that you no longer like that CRAP.

That said, what if there are a few sugary foods that you still want now and again? Maybe you have brunch at a friend's house on Sundays and she makes cannoli that you think are just to die for. The question always comes up, "Can I have some?" Yes. No. Maybe! Here's the deal. Right now, you need to do a full assessment of where you are. And the first question you need to ask yourself is: "Am I at my goal weight?"

If the answer is no, then **now is not the time** to start experimenting with trigger foods and other non–Sugar Savvy solution foods. You need to get to your goal weight to feel the empowerment of what that looks like and feels like! Once you reach your goal weight and have maintained it for at least several weeks, **then** you can start thinking about tweaking your plan.

I'll tell you, once you feel the power that comes from reaching that Fit, Fab, and Fierce weight, you very well may decide that there isn't a damn cookie or cannoli in the universe worth going back for! That's how I feel! I LOVE feeling sexy and energetic and full of life! I know that I get *so* much more out of myself as I age if I take care of myself! I don't want my energy being sucked up thinking about food and having sugar run my life, which is what would happen in my personal case if I tried to go back and have "just one bite." Just one bite and I'm *&&%ed (fill in whatever word works for you!). So I look at that pasta and bread, and to me, it's just cellulite with sauce on it! Those cookies are something that I'd just chew up and slap on my thighs. NO THANK YOU!

It's very hard for you to understand what I'm talking about till you get to your goal weight! You need to get there. Stay there for a bit. THEN make your decisions. You may decide at that point to change your goal weight. You might realize that your original goal weight was unrealistically low; if you're a big-boned gal, you shouldn't aim for to be the same weight as your petite model friend. Conversely, you may originally have been too afraid to set your goal weight low enough, but now you know you can do anything and choose to go for an even lower goal weight. Or, your goal may not be weight-related at all; you may want to reduce your medications or be in less pain or just feel more in control of your eating.

But until you hit that goal weight, I want you to be a little obsessed with eating and thinking and doing things the Sugar Savvy solution way! Re-

The 10 Sugar Savvy Power Points

I've given you a LOT of information here! A lifetime's worth really. It's all very important, but I understand that it might be difficult to keep track of! Some Sugar Savvy Sisters liked to have a quick visual reminder of the basics of Sugar Savvy eating. For them (and maybe you!), I created these 10 Sugar Savvy power points. Make a copy and tack it on your refrigerator as a reminder of your commitment to Sugar Savvy living. (It will also be a helpful reminder for family and friends who visit!)

❶ **Avoid added sugar.** Stay away from sugary treats like candy, cookies, cakes, and other junk foods. Watch out for added sugars in salad dressings, tomato sauces, breakfast cereals, other processed foods, and especially DRINKS! Remember, no more than 24 grams in 24 hours!

❷ **Drink water.** Water is life. Without water, this plan does not work. Drink eight 8-ounce glasses a day.

❸ **Avoid processed foods.** Eat as close to nature as possible! Stay away from food that comes boxed, bagged, wrapped in plastic, and loaded with sugar, salt, additives, and chemicals.

❹ **Eat fruits and especially Vital Veggies!** Enjoy all of nature's best— 2 servings of fruit and 4 or more servings of veggies daily. Eat all the colors of the rainbow: red, yellow, pink, green, purple, orange, and blue . . . even white!

❺ **Go with good grains like our Supercharged Carbs.** Enjoy brown rice, wild rice, millet, barley, quinoa and other whole grains (just keep the serving size

member, you are creating a **new normal** for yourself! Beating addictions, especially when you may not have even known you had them, takes courage and tremendous power.

All that said, once you've hit your goal weight—and maybe, like Perri, you hit it 2 weeks in!—and you find that you still occasionally crave a cup-

(continued on page 144)

to ½ cup or less) unless these prove to be a trigger food for you, in which case you should avoid grains completely.

❻ Enjoy lean protein. Beans, peas, and legumes are good sources of protein, plus fiber and other nutrients. Chicken, turkey, fish, shellfish, pork and occasional cuts of lean red meat, and eggs can also be healthy in small amounts. Stay away from sausage, bacon, processed lunchmeats, fatty marbled beef, and fried meats.

❼ Have calcium-rich foods. Dairy foods are not the only sources of calcium and vitamin D. Try calcium-enriched substitutes such as rice, soy or almond milk, and make sure you get other calcium-rich foods such as dark leafy greens, soybeans, and white beans. If you do choose dairy, stick with fat-free items and always watch for added sugar or salt!

❽ Avoid or limit salt. Do your best to steer clear of salty snacks. Watch out for hidden salts in soups, cheese, packaged rice mixes, soy sauce, and other condiments.

❾ Avoid enriched white flour. Avoid anything made with enriched white flour (especially wheat flour), such as breads, bread crumbs, crackers, baked goods, and regular pastas. Remember, you're always seeking out whole grains!

❿ Go easy on fats. Avoid most saturated and trans fats (those that are solid at room temperature), but do enjoy small portions of healthy fats. A tablespoon or two of olive oil, coconut oil, or other vegetable oil per day is fine, as are the good-for-you fats in fish, avocados, nuts, and seeds.

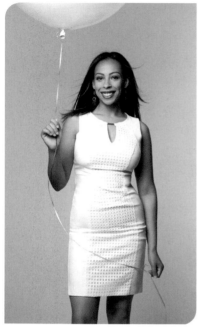

Madeline De La Cruz, Age 22

Madeline was the first Sugar Savvy Sister to reach her goal weight, having **lost a total of 55 pounds** since she first started following Voltage's principles in the Energy Up! program.

Lost 3.8 lbs and 4 inches in 6 weeks!

By the time she was a freshman in high school, Madeline was 190 pounds—the heaviest weight she'd been in her life. "My family members were overweight and I was in an environment where you just ate a lot of carbs and sugar and didn't really think about it. To me, spaghetti and rice was a perfectly fine meal. I just didn't know better at the time," she says.

But Madeline was quick to learn. After being introduced to the Sugar Savvy way of eating through Voltage's Energy Up! program, she started making changes immediately to eliminate added sugar and put more nutrition in her diet. "My weight started to decrease immediately once I started eating Sugar Savvy. Leaving pastries and white rice behind was the hardest part. But I learned to try new foods I'd never had before, especially vegetables."

Madeline's weight dropped steadily until she hit 140, her original goal

> "The more I learn, the more successful I am."

weight. She was happy with how she felt there, but believed she still had room for improvement in her diet. Voltage told her if she pressed forward, she could reach a goal weight of 130 and look and feel amazing. "I didn't want to deprive myself, but I was willing to go for it. I figured there's always room to learn and grow and improve. I started following the formulas and keeping a food diary so I could see exactly what and how much I was eating," she says.

Madeline realized that she wasn't creating well-balanced meals and that her portions tended to be bigger than she needed. "I would have too much protein and carbs, especially plantains and potatoes, and not enough vegetables. The formulas made it easy to always incorporate the right amount of protein, fat, and carbohydrate," she says. "I've also learned that I can occasionally have a cookie or sweet now and it doesn't take over and consume me. Before starting this plan, I would just eat the whole box or bag whenever I started eating. Now I've changed. I don't really want those things anymore and when I do occasionally have a bite of something, it isn't a big deal.

"Following the Sugar Savvy plan also reminded me that I need to exercise more. So I downloaded an app off my iPhone called Moves that tracks your movement, which motivated me to walk much more," she says.

Madeline reached her new goal weight and is so inspired by her transformation, she recently graduated with her bachelor of science in biology and is applying to medical school to become a pediatrician. "I want to take this message out to the children so I can help others lead healthier, Fit, Fab, and Fierce lives."

Madeline's favorite affirmation: I am happy! I am healthy! I am a superstar!

(continued from page 141)

cake or a slice of pizza, that is the time to approach those cravings for those old foods through your new Sugar Savvy eyes and mind-set. When I finish dinner and want a little something sweet, I'm sure as hell not going back to the Cheesecake Factory, but I **have** found various vegan bakeries around New York that use only whole grains and sweeten with agave that make delightful and delicious cupcakes. I would never buy them and bring them back to my home by the dozen, but I would buy and have one and be cool with it. Enough said. I don't like CRAP. Any CRAP! But I love a nutritious, delicious dessert periodically.

> If you get off-track, adopt this mantra: "I forgot **I only want foods** that make me Fit, Fab, and Fierce!"

Sugar Savvy Sister Perri Blumberg also has found that now that she has really changed what she wants, she can really have just one of something. "I'm totally free from not being able to have 'just one' cookie, but I've noticed other bad habits of mine (like binge-watching a whole season of a junky reality TV show in one massive sitting spree) are gone too. I have a much better sense of moderation and just one crummy but oh-so-good episode of *The Bachelor* with just one cookie is totally doable for me now."

If, however, you take a few bites and find yourself unable to stop, that food clearly does not work for you regardless of how nutritionally sound it is. You can keep eating it if you like—but now that you've experienced the pure, natural energy of the Sugar Savvy solution, I'm going to bet you won't want to. We had a number of Sugar Savvy Sisters who found they really couldn't go back to their triggers without having them taking over their lives. So they happily embraced the Sugar Savvy lifestyle without looking back!

"I never really looked at it as a diet or things that I couldn't have," says Aris Pacheco. "When I started really losing so much weight that it was noticeable all my friends and people at work were like, 'Okay. What diet are you on?' because I used to go on diets and tell everyone about it. This time I tell them very honestly, 'I'm not on a diet. I am eating what I want. But I'm just eating different things.' I'm making a lifestyle choice to cook and eat different things because I like how it makes me feel and it's what I want to do." Aris is a sharp Sugar Savvy Sister and nearly 13 pounds lighter because of it!

If you do occasionally go back to a trigger food and binge on it, don't beat yourself up or feel like a loser or even say, "I can't have that food anymore!" The phrase that works for me is: "I forgot I don't like that food. I forgot that food doesn't work for me. I forgot that I only want foods that make me Fit, Fabulous, and Fierce." Then go back to what works! (Remember, you can go back to the Palate Cleanse if you feel like you have gotten far off track.)

No matter where you are on the spectrum, whether you still have a little (or a lot) of weight to lose or whether you've nailed your goal weight, going forward for the rest of your journey, this is not about being PERFECT. It is also not all about numbers on a scale. Weight is certainly one measure of progress and success, but it is not the ONLY one. Some of our Sugar Savvy Sisters are technically still categorized as "obese" according to their body mass index (30 and above). Yet they are healthier than they've ever been. They are off medications. They are full of energy and happy and eating Sugar Savvy. Yes, the weight is still coming off, but they are already successful! ***You can be big but beautiful, healthy, and full of life!*** The Sugar Savvy solution is about always doing the best you can do. If you do your best to stay away from sugary processed foods and eat **real foods**, you will be a Fit, Fab, Fierce Sugar Savvy Sister in no time!

Remember, you are a leader! As you transform, your family and friends will want to follow and you will be able to show them how. As they change, more will change, and eventually the food industry will have to follow US! We are leading the way. DO NOT STOP NOW!!! I am **happy**! I am **healthy**! And I choose to be **powerful and strong** for all to see! Energy Up! *WHOO!!!*

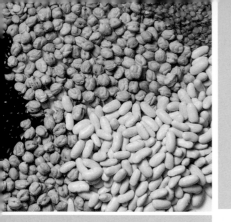
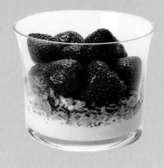
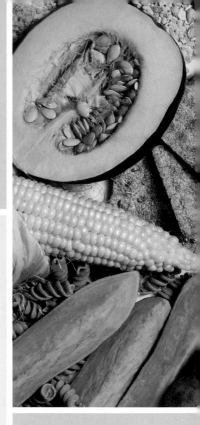
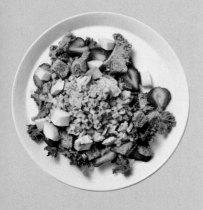
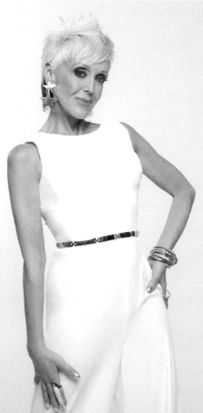
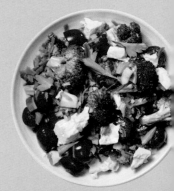
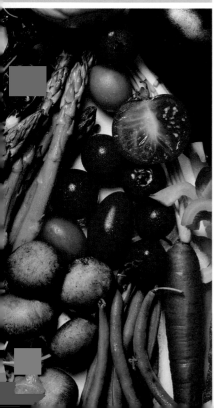
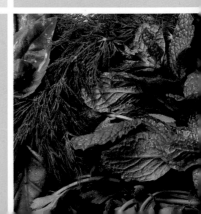
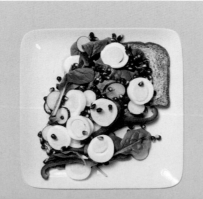

PART 3

THE FIT, FAB, AND FIERCE DETAILS!

Ready to take on the world? You will be after you dig into the AMAZING Sugar Savvy Meal Plan and Workout! Every detail, every nuance, every little thing you need to know, buy, chop, cook, and consume is in here! This is your road map to a Fit, Fab, and Fierce new life! I've shown you the Sugar Savvy solution and once that light goes on, you don't want to live in the dark anymore.

The recipes and routines that follow are the core of the 6-week plan. But they're more than that. They're a reference you can use for the rest of your life! I'm as Sugar Savvy as they come and I'm STILL discovering new foods and combinations of foods through this plan!

I promise this will be the most powerful, yet simple and delicious eating plan you've ever seen, as well as a simple, effective, and energizing workout. Our 17 Sugar Savvy Sisters lost more than 100 pounds after just 3 weeks of following it! By Week 6, they'd shed almost 168 pounds . . . and they continued to lose long afterwards.

CHAPTER 10

THE SUGAR SAVVY MEAL PLAN

Sugar Savvy foods and formulas for sweet success!

"I figured I was doomed from the start because I do not cook. I have never cooked. But here I am cooking! And I love it. I never, ever thought it could be done—a meal plan that is so easy, even I can do it!"

— YOSELIS BALBI, 38,
WHO LOST **15.4 POUNDS** IN **6 WEEKS**

Most Americans blindly eat whatever is served up on the grocery store shelves or restaurant menus by the sugar empire . . . because they don't know better. But now you know! And *once you know, you know.* It's like when I finally got sober after years of being a falling-down drunk. I'm so clear and healthy and energetic there's no going back to the dark! It's time to put boots to the ground and **march toward the light and join the Sugar Savvy Sisterhood!**

> Take back control over food so **food doesn't control you.**

I've told you in great detail what NOT to eat and why. I've told you *how* I want you to eat—Sugar Savvy, the way nature intended. You've cleansed your palate to give your taste buds a break from the daily sugar and salt assault so they can wake up to the more subtle flavors of fresh, whole foods. Now it's time to learn *what* to eat. The Sugar Savvy Meal Plan is the easiest way to enjoy awesome, amazing, live foods that don't have tons of CRAP added in!

I've created this plan with the help of Jessica Issler, a registered dietitian and certified diabetes educator. When I first spoke with Jessica she told me that when she counsels clients, the first thing she tells them is to "take back control over food so food doesn't control you." Amen! To that end, this plan is carefully designed to help you unplug from the Processed Food Matrix and give you a fresh start. *Be forewarned: You will be expected to cook!* I've always eaten very healthy foods. But I will confess that in the past I would buy my Sugar Savvy foods and not put much effort into meal preparation beyond eating them raw or blending them into soups. Well, to the shock of everyone who knows me, Jessica helped me get cooking and I am loving it! I have discovered that it's so much easier than I ever imagined. And the food is FANTASTIC!

Yes, it will take some time and energy at first, but once you get the hang of it, it takes no time at all! While we're talking about time, let me tell you something. The Sugar Savvy Sisters, not to mention the hundreds of students and clients I've worked with for the past 30 years, used to waste a ton of it obsessing about food, bingeing and then starving themselves, dieting and beating themselves up, all because they're addicted to the CRAP the food industry calls **"convenient"**! It is NOT convenient to be constantly preoccupied with cookies and chips. It is NOT convenient to eat a full meal only to be tired and hungry 2 hours later. It is NOT convenient to go to a posse of doctors for your heart meds, diabetes care, arthritis pain, and other sickness because your "convenient" diet is slowly killing you. There is NOTHING convenient about convenience foods! They are a NIGHTMARE we must wake up from.

A FORMULA FOR SUCCESS

Because it is designed to educate you and sharpen your eating intuition, the Sugar Savvy Meal Plan is going to be like none other you've ever seen. We intentionally avoided telling you exactly what to eat every day for 30 days (though we have provided plenty of examples for you to follow, if you find that easier). Instead, Jessica has created Power Meal formulas that will help you build balanced, nutritious, and yes, delicious Sugar Savvy meals!

Eventually, your intuition will take over and you will automatically say, "I need a little of this and a little of that and a LOT of that—vegetables!—to make my meal." But in the meantime, Jessica has taken the guesswork out of it for you and created a blueprint that clearly outlines how many servings of each food group you need to pack in maximum nutrition and stay satisfied and craving free. Remember, the goal is to rewire the way your brain thinks about food and to retrain your taste buds to enjoy real, whole, natural food.

The first step is exploring the huge variety of foods that are naturally Sugar Savvy. All too often, when people hear me talk about adding more fresh vegetables to their diets, they think they'll be condemned to a lifetime of lettuce and tomatoes. But take another look when you're at the grocery store. What are those vibrant bunches of leafy greens sitting next to the pale heads of iceberg? Never tried kale, collard greens, or arugula? Now's the time! And what about jicama or kohlrabi? Don't worry if you can't pronounce them; you can eat them! Nor are you limited to the produce department. Meat and poultry are still on the menu, if you desire, as are nuts, cheeses, whole grains, and more. You just might want to try different forms of your favorite foods (buckwheat noodles instead of regular spaghetti, for instance) and learn new ways of cooking with them (hint—keep preparation methods simple and portions petite). But, as I've been saying all along, Sugar Savvy eating is DELISH; I eat more food now than I ever did when I was bingeing on cookies. Of course, you're not going to love every food. But I promise you'll have a lot of fun trying new foods—and you never know what's going to become your new favorite.

Note: Any change—even a healthy one!—in your diet (meaning, an increase or decrease in different foods, beverages, herbs, supplements, or nutrients) can interfere with some medications. So check with your healthcare provider before starting the plan. Also, a significant increase in fiber (from your Sugar Savvy veggies, whole grains, and beans) can cause some digestive discomfort at first. To prevent this, be extra vigilant about getting your 8 glasses of water per day. It may also help to cook more of your vegetables instead of eating them raw. Or start with a smaller amount of fiber-rich foods and gradually ramp up.

SUGAR SAVVY FOOD GROUPS

Here are the food groups you'll be mixing and matching to make your Sugar Savvy meals and drinks.

These are similar to the food groups you learned in school, but Jessica and I have categorized some foods differently and have highlighted those from each group we feel are particularly healthy. In general, these foods are grouped according to their macronutrient profile; that is, how much and what type of nutrients they provide per serving. You may think of low-fat cheese, for example, as a "dairy food." But in the Sugar Savvy Meal Plan, you'll find it under Proteins because that's the primary macronutrient it provides. Beans, peas, and legumes contain protein, too, but also have naturally occurring starch. Because their nutritional makeup per serving is different, we put them in a category all their own.

It's important to note also that the food lists below are not exhaustive, meaning there are foods we haven't listed that may fit into each group. These are just some of my favorites! The serving sizes listed here are approximate, based on the estimated calories, fat, carbohydrate, and protein you can expect to find in the foods listed. When you first start following the Sugar Savvy Meal Plan, I suggest that you weigh and measure out your foods to get a sense of the amount we're talking about (especially for proteins and grains, which we tend to overeat). But after the first couple of weeks, there is no need to be so exact. And you never need to count calories or grams of carbohydrate, fat, or protein. Jessica has done that math for you so the only thing you do count on the Sugar Savvy plan is sugar grams! And if you follow the meal plan, you don't even really need to worry about going over the limit!

SUGAR SAVVY FOOD GROUPS AT A GLANCE	
Food Group	Examples of Foods Included
Veggies	Leafy greens; nonstarchy vegetables
Carbs	100% whole grains and whole grain products, such as sprouted grain breads and pastas; starchy vegetables, such as potatoes and winter squash
Fruits	Whole fruits
Proteins	Tofu, tempeh, low-fat cheeses, eggs, lean meat, fish, poultry
Fats	Healthy oils, nuts, seeds
Beans & Peas	Beans, peas, legumes
Milks & Yogurt	Milk, yogurt, fortified nondairy milks

Veggies: Leafy Greens and Nonstarchy Vegetables

These low-calorie nutrition powerhouses are high in fiber, water and a host of vitamins and minerals, all of which are vital for a Fit, Fab, and Fierce you. As you'll see, no matter what meal formulas you choose, veggies will often outnumber or outweigh the other food on your plate. It's almost impossible to overeat vegetables—that's why, as you'll see, Vital Veggies form one of the Power Bases for our formulas. You'll note that starchy veggies like potatoes are categorized as carbs, because they have a higher carb count than nonstarchy vegetables.

Just remember that less is more when preparing veggies. Stick to fresh produce or plain frozen vegetables, and serve them raw, lightly steamed, boiled, roasted, or lightly sautéed in a small amount of healthy oil. Avoid canned veggies that have been loaded up with sodium, or veggies cooked in butter or creamy sauces until they are dead, dead, dead. When creating any Sugar Savvy meal, include a wide range of colorful veggie varieties to get the most disease-fighting bang for your buck! Eat the colors of the rainbow! And eat vegetables in season—this will not only help ensure that you get the variety of nutrients you need, but it's also less expensive.

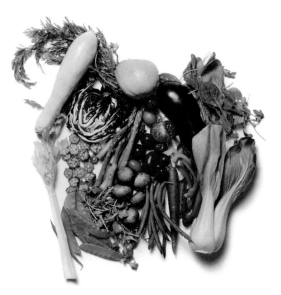

VEGGIES

For all vegetables listed below, the serving size is 1 cup raw or ½ cup cooked.

Leafy Greens

Arugula	Mesclun
Bok choy	Mustard greens
Cabbage: red, green, Napa, Savoy, etc.	Radicchio
Collard greens	Spinach
Endive	Spring greens
Escarole	Swiss chard
Kale	Turnip greens
Lettuce: red, green, Bibb, etc.	Watercress

Nonstarchy Vegetables

Artichoke	Mushrooms
Asparagus	Okra
Beets	Onions
Broccoli	Parsnips
Brussels sprouts	Peppers
Carrots	Radishes
Cauliflower	Rutabaga
Celery	Shallots
Cucumber	Snow peas or sugar snap peas
Fennel	Summer squash
Green beans	Turnips
Eggplant	Tomato
Green onions (scallions)	Water chestnut
Kohlrabi	Zucchini
Leeks	

Note: Choose organic if possible.

Carbs: 100 Percent Whole Grains and Starchy Vegetables

Carbs can be problematic. Sugar, after all, is a carb—and we all know by now what too much sugar can do to us! But not all carbs are alike. Whole grains and starchy vegetables provide carbs the way nature intended: full of fiber, antioxidants, and other nutrients to help fuel our bodies and our minds. It is crucial that you choose Sugar Savvy carbs—what I like to call Supercharged Carbs. In this group you will find starchy vegetables, grains, and grain-based foods that you can swap for one another. So if any foods in this category tend to be a trigger for you—say, pasta—you can get similar nutrition and satisfaction from another source, such as barley, corn, quinoa, or winter squash.

Starchy vegetables include potatoes, winter squash, and yams. You can't go wrong with these (unless any turn out to be a trigger food for you). Likewise, we have suggested a wide array of whole grains, including some, ranging from amaranth to wheat berries, you may never have heard of but will certainly learn to love. The great thing about these is that they're not processed so you won't have to pore over a label to determine if it is a whole grain.

What about breads, crackers, pastas, and the like? **If any of these is a trigger food for you, stay away from it for the duration of the 6-week plan.** Stick with some of the alternatives listed on page 158. If grains are not trigger foods for you, just be sure to read the labels to make sure you're getting whole grains! Take a look at the ingredient list and be sure that each grain has the word "whole" in front of it. Here are a few examples of what to look for:

- whole grain _____
- whole _____
- stone-ground whole _____

Some exceptions to this rule: Brown rice and oats or oatmeal are whole grains even though it may not always say "whole" in the ingredient list.

What about sprouted grains? Sprouted grains are whole grains that have just started to sprout, or grow into a plant. The sprouts are ground up and used to make grain-based products like bread, pasta, and tortillas. Many believe that the sprouting process makes the nutrients in the grain more easily digestible and more information is starting to emerge regarding additional health benefits. We love them for their hearty taste as well! You can find them in the freezer section of most grocery stores.

As a general rule of thumb, choose foods that have the shortest ingredient lists! There'll be less chance of unhealthy stuff being added in *and* less for you to examine to determine if you're getting it right! And, of course, it's very important to remember your sugar-sleuthing skills: Make sure there is no added sugar (in any form) on the ingredients label, nor excess salt, unhealthy fat, or other unwanted ingredients.

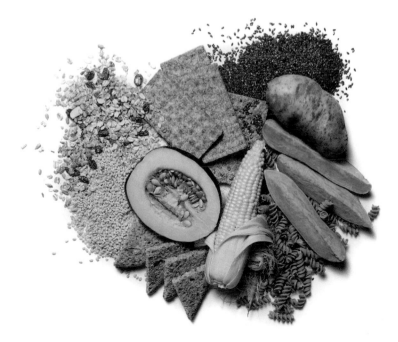

CARBS

In general, the serving size for most carbs listed is ½ cup cooked.

Whole Grains	Serving Size
Amaranth*	½ cup cooked
Barley (hulled or "hull-less"—not pearled)	½ cup cooked
Brown, red, purple, or black rice*	⅓ cup cooked
Buckwheat*	½ cup cooked
Bulgur	½ cup cooked
Corn*	½ cup cooked
Farro	½ cup cooked
Kamut	½ cup cooked
Millet*	½ cup cooked
Oats*	½ cup cooked
Quinoa*	½ cup cooked
Rye, or rye berries	½ cup cooked
Spelt	½ cup cooked
Teff*	½ cup cooked
Wheat berries	½ cup cooked
Wild rice*	½ cup cooked
Whole Grain Products	**Serving Size**
Sprouted whole grain and 100% whole grain bread, tortillas, English muffins, bagels, buns, etc. (no sugar added)	1–2 slices (or the amount that contains ~15 grams of carbohydrate)
Sprouted whole grain and 100% whole grain pasta (no sugar added) such as buckwheat (soba), quinoa, or brown rice noodles	½ cup cooked
Muesli (grain portion must be 100% whole grain with no sugar added)	¼ cup
100% whole grain, high-fiber, nut- or seed-based crackers (no sugar added and low in sodium)	Varies (the amount that contains ~15 grams of carbohydrate)
Starchy Vegetables	**Serving Size**
Spaghetti squash*	1½ cups cooked
Sweet potatoes*	½ cup cooked
White potatoes*	½ cup cooked
Winter squash (acorn, butternut, kabocha)*	1 cup cooked
Yams*	½ cup cooked

Note: Foods marked with an asterisk above are naturally gluten free and generally safe for people with celiac disease or gluten sensitivity to eat. But be aware of possible contaminants in processing.

If you're new to cooking with whole grains, keep in mind that these are as different from your old, dead carbs as fresh produce is from mushy canned vegetables. I forgot to warn our Sugar Savvy Sisters about this when I gave them all a box of Kamut to try. An ancient grain that looks like rice, Kamut is meant to have a chewy, al dente texture that gives a bit of crunch when you eat it. One of our sisters cooked it three times, letting it simmer away more than 2 hours, thinking it was supposed to get mushy like white rice. When it never did, she assumed she'd done something wrong and pitched the whole batch!

Once she knew what to expect, though, it opened up a whole new world of eating filled with lively textures to mix and match. That's the idea here! Remember, we are creating a **new normal**. Once you get a taste for these exciting, nutritious powerhouses, you'll never go back to mushy dead food again!

> Once you get a taste for these exciting, **nutritious powerhouses,** you'll never go back to eating mushy dead food again!

Fruits: Fresh and Dried Fruits (no sugar added)

Like veggies, fruits pack a nutritional punch in the form of vitamins, minerals, antioxidants, fiber, and water, but they have more calories due to their naturally occurring sugar. This does not make them bad foods or take them off our plan. You will see fruits called for in some of our Power Meal formulas, and they're an ingredient in all of our Power Drinks as well. You need about 2 servings from this food group a day.

As we saw in Chapter 2, most commercially available fruit juices are LOADED with shocking amounts of added sugar. But even if you make juice yourself at home, you are breaking down much of the fiber that helps slow down and rein in the fruit's naturally occurring sugars. So it's always best to go with the "real deal" here—whole fruit (in the appropriate amounts) rather than juice.

Dried fruits can be a healthy choice, as well; just be sure to get those that don't have any added sugar and stick to the serving sizes listed. It's also important to note that for some people, dried fruit can really be like "nature's candy"—and not in a good way! Because they are so chewy and sweet, dried fruits like raisins and dried apricot slices may be a trigger food for

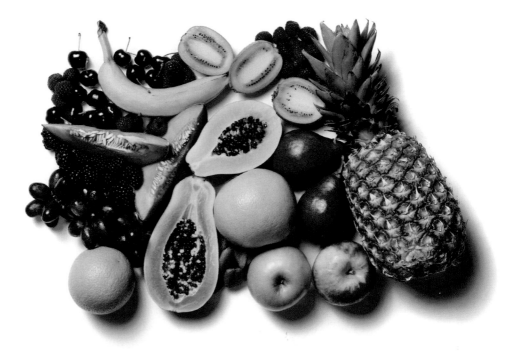

some people. **If you are one of them, then steer clear of dried fruits** for the duration of the 6-week Sugar Savvy solution and just stick to fresh fruits.

As with veggies, frozen fruits with no sugar added can also be a good alternative, but beware of canned fruits, especially those labeled "canned in syrup"—*syrup* is just another word for added sugar! And again, make it a habit to eat in season. Fruit that's in season will be fresher, taste better, and be less expensive than fruit that's not. Plus, this is an easy and delicious way to ensure that you get a variety of nutrients.

FRUITS

In general, the serving size for fresh fruit is 1 piece (about 2–3 inches in diameter) or ½–1 cup.

Fresh Fruit	Serving Size
Whole fruits such as apples, pears, peaches, nectarines, oranges	1 (about 2½–3 in. in diameter) or about 1 cup slices
Berries such as blackberries, blueberries, cranberries, raspberries, sliced strawberries	About 1 cup
Melons such as cantaloupe, honeydew, watermelon	About 1 cup cubed
Tropical fruits such as guava, mango, papaya, pineapple	About ¾ cup chunks or cubes
Small fruits such as figs, kiwifruit, plums	2 (about 1½–2 in. in diameter)
Bananas	1 (about 6 in. long) or ½ cup slices
Grapes	15–20 (about ½ cup)
Pomegranate	½ cup arils (seeds)
Dried Fruit	**Serving Size**
Apples	4 rings or ¼ cup
Apricots	¼ cup halves
Cranberries	3 Tbsp
Figs	3
Goji berries	¼ cup
Medjool dates	3
Prunes	3 whole
Raisins	2 Tbsp

Note: Choose organic if possible.

Proteins: Lean Meats, Vegetarian Proteins, Low-Fat Cheeses, and Eggs

When I need to charge my batteries and get my ENERGY UP, protein is the first place I turn in my diet. It fuels my muscles like nothing else, probably because it literally *becomes* my muscles! The protein that we eat gets digested and absorbed into our bodies as amino acids. Amino acids, in turn, become the "building blocks" for our bodies. So to truly look and feel Fit, Fab, and Fierce, it's important to get enough protein—and to get it from a variety of sources, so we get all the amino acids we need.

But, of course, you want to avoid bringing sugar or any of its evil sidekicks along for the ride. Not many protein-rich foods contain naturally occurring or added sugar (with the exception of milks and yogurts, which are in their own food group), but some of the condiments you usually use on meat, such as barbecue sauce and ketchup, do. In addition, most red meat is loaded with saturated fat and certain preparation methods (such as frying) add a lot of unhealthy fat. Another big issue is sodium, especially in some deli meats, sausages, bacon, and meatballs. These "processed" meats are also often full of artificial additives and preservatives like nitrites.

So in our protein food group you'll find lean cuts of red meat, pork,

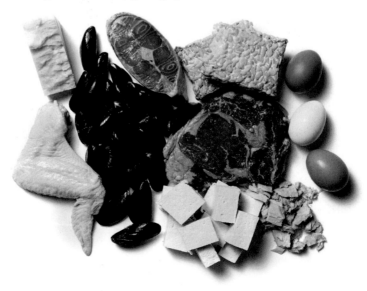

poultry, fish, cheese, and eggs. And try vegetarian proteins like tofu or tempeh; you'll be surprised at how versatile they are.

At first, you may be tempted to exclaim, "Where's the beef?!" We've gotten used to great big slabs of meat on our plate, but that usually adds up to more than we really need (unless we're training for the Olympics). Day to day, anywhere from 10 to 35 percent of our calories (about 50 to 150 grams for the average adult woman) can come from protein. We suggest aiming for around 15 to 20 percent most of the time. For reference, a McDonald's Double Quarter Pounder with Cheese has 48 grams of protein, enough to meet the USDA's Recommended Daily Allowance of 46 grams.

You may have heard the recommendation to keep your meat portions to

PROTEINS

The serving size for meats is for the cooked portion trimmed of all visible fat.

Vegetarian Proteins	Serving Size
Tempeh	1–2 oz (or the amount that contains ~7 grams of protein)
Tofu	1–3 oz (or the amount that contains ~7 grams of protein)
Low-Fat Cheeses and Eggs	**Serving Size**
Cheese (about 3 g fat per oz)	1 oz
Cottage cheese (low fat, no sodium added)	¼ cup
Eggs	1 large
Lean Meats, Fish, and Poultry	**Serving Size**
Beef: tenderloin, sirloin, round, roast, flank steak	1 oz
Fish, fresh or frozen; canned tuna (light, reduced-sodium, packed in water)	1 oz
Pork: tenderloin, boneless loin chops	1 oz
Poultry: chicken, turkey, etc. (no skin)	1 oz
Shellfish	1 oz

Note: Choose organic meats when possible, as well as grass-fed beef and wild-caught fish. In the case of vegetarian proteins, choose non-GMO organic products made from whole soy beans that are fortified with calcium, vitamin D, and, ideally, vitamin B12.

the size of a deck of cards. That is equivalent to about 2 to 3 ounces of meat, and is certainly a more reasonable portion than a double burger or a steak. But for the duration of the 6-week Sugar Savvy plan, while you're rewiring the way your brain thinks about food, we're asking you to use 1 ounce of meat as a serving (some meals call for 2 servings). But since you'll be mixing and matching protein sources (so that you're getting protein from beans and peas, milks and yogurts, and even whole grains, as well as from meat and eggs), you'll be balancing out your 1 to 2 ounces of grilled chicken or your 1- to 2-egg omelette with so many other healthy foods, it won't seem skimpy at all.

So as part of your new normal, I want you to **start thinking of meat as a condiment or as a side dish** to all the delicious Vital Veggies and other Sugar Savvy foods you're enjoying. You may even be inspired to go meat free, or even vegan. If you do, just make sure you are getting enough vitamin B12 and eat a variety of protein-containing foods daily.

Portion Shock Exercise

Portions are **_astronomically out of control_** in our country. Though you are eating a lot of food on the Sugar Savvy Meal Plan, the portions of starchy carbs and protein foods are more appropriate—and likely smaller than your eyes have become accustomed to seeing on your plate. I would very much like you to get measuring cups (liquid and dry) and a food scale for this plan (you can buy them at retailers like Walmart or Target for less than $25). Not that I want you to be weighing every morsel that goes into your mouth for the rest of your life, but you MUST get a handle on what real, appropriate portions look like. I mean, look around. Do you think we've been eating the RIGHT AMOUNTS? Not on your life! This is true even of fruit, which can be very easy to overeat. (It never occurs to many people that an extra large banana can be almost like eating three bananas!) Some of the Sugar Savvy Sisters were really stressed out about this

Fats: Healthy Oils, Nuts, Seeds, and Other Healthy Fats

Yes, it's true: Too much dietary fat—one of sugar's notorious evil sidekicks—can cause a host of health problems, but we really do need fat in our diet! Certainly, you should avoid nasty trans and saturated fats, like those found in fast-food burgers, many packaged pastries, some margarines, chips, and other snack foods containing hydrogenated or partially hydrogenated oils. Instead, focus on healthy monosaturated and polyunsaturated fats found in the foods listed on page 166 (like seeds and nuts).

One notable exception to the saturated fat rule: The type of saturated fat in coconut oil may be beneficial for weight loss—plus, it's an AMAZING body oil! I not only eat coconut oil, I use it as a moisturizer and to make my hair shine!

at first. But then they realized that they could load up on veggies and, in fact, **they were full on less food**. "When I saw the portions, I thought, wow, that's not a lot of food . . . it's nothing!" noted Bonnie O'Gallagher. "But then I started snacking on veggies and quickly saw I really didn't need that much food to be full!" That's right. They weren't stuffed like you would be after an all-you-can-eat (but really don't need to eat) buffet. But they were genuinely satisfied!

So put your typical portion on the scale or in the cup and and see how many ounces that piece of meat or serving of pasta really is. You'll be shocked! We are so used to having 5, 6, maybe even 7 or 8 servings piled on our plates! At first, it might look measly to dish out the correct amount, but **try it**. You really don't need that much food. You're going to change, so you'll feel stuffed and gross when you gorge yourself on the portions you used to eat. Trust me. Just like what you want to eat is going to change, how much you want to eat is going to change as well.

FATS

Healthy Oils	Serving Size
Avocado oil	1 tsp
Coconut oil	1 tsp
Flaxseed oil	1 tsp
Olive oil	1 tsp
Peanut oil	1 tsp
Safflower oil	1 tsp
Sesame oil	1 tsp
Nuts	**Serving Size**
Almonds	8
Cashews	6
Nut butters such as peanut, cashew, and almond butter (natural, no sugar added)	1½ tsp
Peanuts	10
Walnuts	4 halves
Seeds	**Serving Size**
Chia seeds	1 Tbsp
Flaxseed meal	2 Tbsp
Hemp seeds (shelled)	1 Tbsp
Pumpkin seeds	1 Tbsp
Sesame seeds	1 Tbsp
Sunflower seeds	1 Tbsp
Other Healthy Fats	**Serving Size**
Avocado	¼ avocado or 2 Tbsp, diced or mashed
Black olives	8 large
Cacao nibs	1 Tbsp
Coconut milk, light	Varies (the amount that contains ~5 grams of fat)
Green olives	10 large
Hemp milk	¾ cup
Shredded unsweetened coconut	2 Tbsp
Tahini (sesame butter)	2 tsp

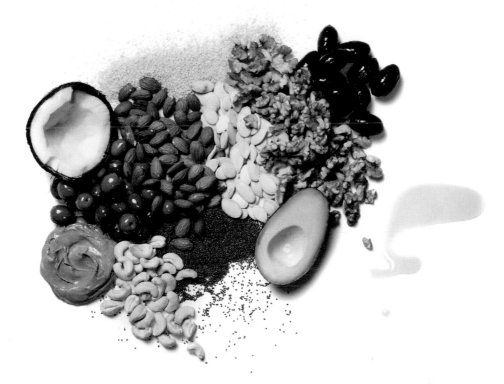

Beans & Peas: Beans, Peas, and Legumes

Beans and peas not only provide you with energy from healthy carbohydrates, they are also all great sources of protein and dietary fiber—all necessary nutrients to fuel your body. This is a three-for-the-price-of-one deal that you should NOT pass up! Including beans in your Power Meals may require a little advance planning (especially if you choose dried beans or legumes), but it is well worth it. If you would like to use canned beans, that is fine, just be sure to buy low-sodium versions and soak and rinse them very well to remove the added sodium that's in the liquid they are usually packed in. Also, choose cans labeled BPA-free when possible. (BPA or bisphenol-A is a chemical in the lining of cans that may contribute to health issues.)

BEANS, PEAS, AND LEGUMES

	Serving Size
Black beans	½ cup cooked
Black-eyed peas	½ cup cooked
Chickpeas (also known as garbanzo beans)	½ cup cooked
Green peas	1 cup cooked
Kidney beans	½ cup cooked
Lima beans	½ cup cooked
Lentils	½ cup cooked
Navy beans	½ cup cooked
Pinto beans	½ cup cooked
Split peas	½ cup cooked
White beans	½ cup cooked

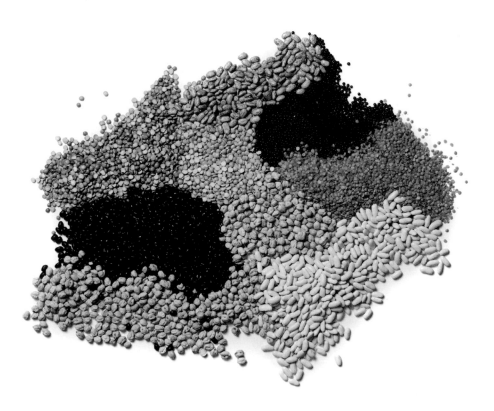

Milks & Yogurt: Milk, Yogurt, and Calcium-Fortified Nondairy Milks

Another group that gives you a mix of macronutrients (protein, carbohydrate, and a little bit of fat in some cases), the milks and yogurt group also offers another key mineral: calcium. And let's not forget its partner, vitamin D. Both are essential for strong bones and good health—plus research shows they can help you lose weight!

Of course, some of the foods we included here are not true "milks" from an animal, but Jessica and I grouped them together because they offer you similar nutrition (mostly protein and some naturally occurring sugar). Just make sure the brands you choose are unsweetened. In the case of milk alternatives like soy milk, almond milk, and rice milk, choose those that have around 8 grams of protein per serving and have been fortified with calcium and vitamins D and B12. Women between the ages of 19 and 50 should be getting 1,000 milligrams of calcium daily, per the USDA's Recommended Dietary Allowance; those over age 50 should get 1,200 milligrams/day. You can get nearly half of that in just 1 cup of fortified soy milk. Other foods from greens to fish are great sources of calcium, but we'll talk more about them later!

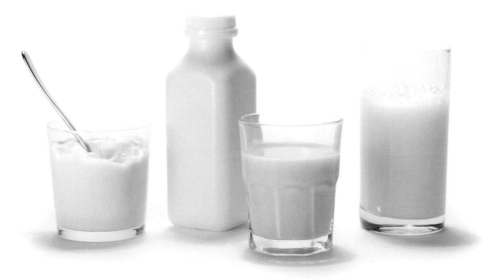

MILKS & YOGURT	
	Serving Size
Skim milk	1 cup (8 oz)
Unsweetened almond milk (fortified with calcium, vitamins D and B12, and added protein)	1 cup (8 oz)
Unsweetened soy milk (made from whole soy beans) (fortified with calcium and vitamins D and B12)	1 cup (8 oz)
Fat-free plain yogurt or plain Greek yogurt (which is higher in protein)	¾ cup (6 oz) (or the amount that contains ~8 grams of protein)
Plain, unsweetened soy yogurt (made from whole soy beans)	¾ cup (6 oz) (or the amount that contains ~8 grams of protein)

Note: Choose organic when possible. For nondairy milks, choose non-GMO products.

Sugar Savvy High-Wattage Foods

While you could certainly make a case for other foods to qualify as super-nutritious, these High-Wattage foods are my faves! Start with the ones you know. Then be adventurous and try something new! **Try to eat at least one a day.** (Jessica has already included them in many of the Power Meals in Chapter 11.) Most are available in the organic or specialty food aisles in your grocery store. If not, check health food stores like Vitamin Shoppe, Whole Foods, or even large retailers like Target or Walmart.

Food	Serving Size	Food Group
Avocado	¼ avocado or 2 Tbsp, diced or mashed	Fats
Bee pollen	1 tsp	Other
Black beans	½ cup cooked	Beans & Peas
Blueberries	1 cup	Fruits
Cacao nibs	¼ cup or 2 Tbsp	Fats
Chia seeds	1 Tbsp	Fats
Flaxseed meal	2 Tbsp	Fats
Garlic	1 tsp or 1 clove	Other
Jalapeño peppers	1 pepper	Veggies
Sweet potatoes	½ cup cooked	Carbs
Unsweetened almond milk (fortified with calcium, vitamins D and B12, and added proten)	1 cup (8 oz)	Milks & Yogurt

FIT, FAB, AND FLAVORFUL FOODS!

Remember, all those years of beating down your taste buds with sugar and salt have desensitized your palate. Now we're bringing it back to life! I promise you that once you start following the Sugar Savvy Meal Plan, your taste buds will be more wide awake and alert than ever and you will savor a whole world of flavors you've been missing! Here are some ideas on how to do that without sabotaging your new normal.

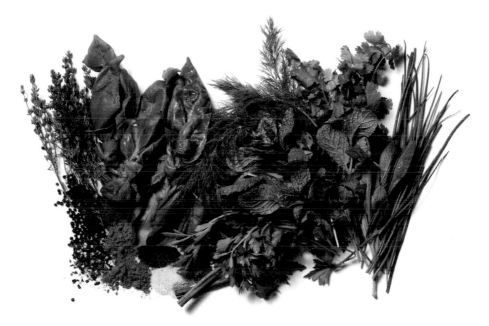

Sugar Savvy Herbs and Spices

Not sugar, but SPICE makes everything nice! Try some of the amazing herbs and spices listed on the next page to brighten up and add zing to your Sugar Savvy meals. Add as much or as little as you'd like! In keeping with the Sugar Savvy philosophy, I prefer to buy fresh herbs whenever possible. I'd even recommend starting a little herb garden in your windowsill! However, you most certainly can use the dried varieties, as they are convenient and have a longer shelf life.

- Allspice
- Basil
- Bay leaves (these are great for adding flavor to dishes; remove before eating)
- Black pepper
- Cardamom
- Chili powder
- Chives
- Cilantro
- Cinnamon
- Cloves
- Cumin
- Dill
- Garlic and garlic powder
- Ginger
- Herbs de Provence
- Hot red pepper flakes
- Mint
- Nutmeg
- Onion powder
- Oregano
- Paprika
- Parsley
- Rosemary
- Sage
- Thyme
- Turmeric
- Yellow curry powder

Sugar Savvy Condiments

As you've seen (and likely have been shocked to see!), popular condiments like ketchup, salad dressing, barbecue sauce, and the like are minefields full of sugar bombs! But that doesn't mean you have to eat your salads and sandwiches naked. Try these Sugar Savvy–approved condiments that will add loads of flavor without adding sugar and unwanted calories. Use as much as you like!

- Apple cider vinegar, such as Bragg's
- Dijon mustard
- Ground red pepper
- Hot sauce (be sure to choose the lowest-sodium option, such as Tabasco)
- Salsa (no sugar added, lowest sodium you can find, such as Muir Glen)

In addition, there are a few condiments I recommend that you use sparingly, as they will add a few calories—too many to fit easily into the Power Meal formulas if you have more than the amount recommended below:

- Marinara sauce (low-sodium and sugar-free, such as Rao's): Use less than ½ cup.

- Nutritional yeast (such as Bragg's): Use 1 Tbsp. Sprinkle it on steamed veggies or popcorn for a "cheesy" flavor.

- Vegenaise Dressing & Sandwich Spread: Use less than 2 tsp. Vegenaise is usually found in the refrigerated section near tofu, tempeh, and meat substitutes.

One more great swap to tell you about: Bragg's Liquid Amino's. Use these instead of soy sauce and get great flavor without added preservatives and ingredients. Just soybeans and water . . . BUT it is a concentrated source of sodium so use sparingly (½ tsp or less).

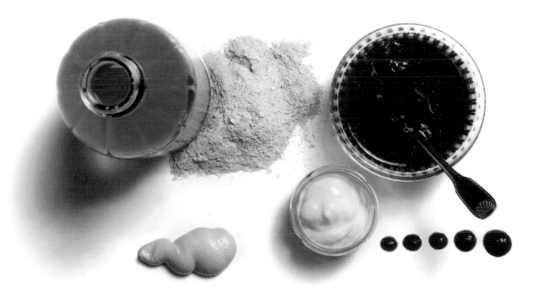

Sugar Savvy–Approved Sweeteners

Now that you've reset your taste buds, you will probably find that treats you used to love taste unbearably sweet. That said, there may still be times when you want to sweeten things up a bit. The sweeteners below are some of my favorites. Some have a little nutrition to offer you along with the sweet taste. When using these sweeteners, you must count the grams of sugar they provide to stay Sugar Savvy. Remember: **no more than 24 grams in 24 hours!**

	Serving Size	Approximate Grams of Sugar per Serving
Agave nectar	1 tsp	5 g
Coconut palm sugar	1 tsp	4 g
Honey	1 tsp	6 g
Maple syrup (100% pure)	1 tsp	4 g
Molasses	1 tsp	5 g
Stevia/Truvia/Nectresse	1 tsp/1 packet	These products actually have zero grams of sugar per serving. We've included them here because they have natural origins.

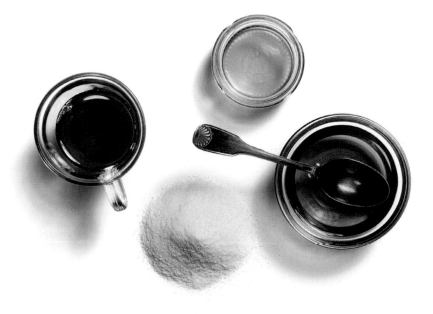

THE SUGAR SAVVY POWER MEALS

Now that you've retrained your mind and your eyes to recognize real, yummy Sugar Savvy foods and maybe even brought home a few bags full of foods you've never tried before, I bet you're wondering what to do with all of them. Enter the Power Meal formulas. I asked Jessica to create these 9 simple "recipes" to help you use all your exciting new Sugar Savvy foods in nutritious mini-meals that will keep you energized and satisfied all day long.

For each of the formulas on pages 178-184, flip back to the food groups depicted by the icon and choose any of the foods in the corresponding chart. This is a delicious, flexible way to create meals with your favorite foods.

Your meals are going to start with one of two Power Bases: Vital Veggies or Supercharged Carbs. These two food groups will form the foundation of your diet. Vital Veggies are a no-brainer: Everyone knows veggies are great for you, so move them over from their normal "side" position and get them front and center on your plate!

You might be a little surprised, though, to see carbs given such a prominent place in the Sugar Savvy Meal Plan. Carbs, as you've learned, have gotten a bad rap because there are a ton of really unhealthy carbs out there . . . such as sugary cereals, white bread, and of course my old nemesis, cookies— all loaded with added sugar! But you, my Sugar Savvy Sisters, are in for a real treat! Real, unprocessed grains and delicious starchy vegetables, like sprouted or 100% whole grain products, quinoa, and sweet potatoes, are not only bursting with nutrients but also with flavor! In making these Supercharged Carbs one of your Power Bases, we are aiming to ***change your idea of what carbs are***. But don't get carried away! Because Supercharged Carbs are more calorically dense, you're going to start small here. Full disclosure: Your Sugar Savvy pasta or rice dish is going to look A LOT different from the one you are used to, but you do still get to enjoy those foods if you want them. As always, though, remember that if any of these foods are a trigger for you, steer clear of them for the duration of the 6-week plan.

Once you've chosen your Power Base, pick a formula to follow. All the formulas start with a reasonable portion of good-for-you fat to help you stay full and feel fabulous. Then choose what protein you're in the mood for. As you'll see, you can choose pure proteins (such as eggs, tofu, fish, or poultry), beans and peas (which provide both protein and carbohydrates), milks or yogurt (which also give you both protein and carbohydrates), or a mix, depending on what you feel like eating that day. Finally, each formula rounds out your meal with either some fruit or added veggies or carbs—all of which come from our Sugar Savvy food groups.

> Aim to get as many colors as possible to get more **health-boosting bang** for you back!

The focus here is not on eliminating any one type of food or food group (except, of course, added sugar or any trigger foods) but instead on putting healthy foods together in appropriate proportions. Many of us tend to eat way too much protein, unhealthy carbs, and nasty fats and not enough veggies and fruit. This plan aims to fix that. Again, this is about changing the way we look at meal planning and preparation. Let's not plan each night's dinner around what meat is on sale at the supermarket. Instead, let's open our pantry and grab some brown rice or some new and exciting grains like farro and millet and think, *"What can I put with this to make a Sugar Savvy Meal?"* Sometimes it might be lean meat, veggies, and healthy fats, but other times, let's make it beans or vegetarian proteins. Variety is the spice of life, after all!

Vital Veggie Power Meals

Leafy greens and nonstarchy vegetables form one of our Power Bases because you can essentially add anything to them and you've got a fantastic meal! Your Vital Veggie Power Base consists of 2 servings of veggies—you can mix and match any combination of veggies for this, but Jessica and I do suggest including both leafy greens and nonstarchy vegetables every day.

Choose nutrient- and pigment-rich greens such as kale, baby spinach, and arugula to build your leafy green portion of this Power Base. (Paler greens such as iceberg lettuce are "low-wattage" choices that don't have much to offer you from a nutritional—or taste—standpoint). Add in one or several more nonstarchy vegetables to round out this Power Base; aim to get in as many colors as possible to get more health-boosting bang for your buck! The key here is to get a VARIETY! (If you find it easier to prepare a meal with 2 servings of all one vegetable—or just really feel like loading up on lots of curly green kale—that's okay. What's important is that you vary what veggies you eat over the course of a day, or even a week, to make sure you get a variety of different nutrients.)

Note that a significant increase in fiber can sometimes cause a little excess gas or other digestive discomfort at first. The best way to prevent this? Drink your water! Also, I suggest sticking with Power Meals made of cooked, rather than raw, veggies. If your stomach is really bothering you, start with a smaller amount of vegetables at first and gradually ramp up to the full 2 servings per meal.

With each of the formulas below, you will start with your Vital Veggie Power Base and then add 1 Fat. After that, it's all about the protein you want. Are you in the mood for fish? Want to top your salad with cottage cheese? Would you like some eggs? Then you will use the Pure Protein formula to round out your meal. Want to use up some of the beans, peas, or legumes you have on hand? Then check out the Mean Bean formula. Not sure you want to limit yourself to protein from just one group? Then the Mix It Up formula is the way to go. Following the formula to build your meal will help to ensure that you get the right amount of total energy and a balance of macronutrients each and every time. Check out Chapter 11 for some examples of actual meals made from these formulas.

Pure Protein

Start with: Vital Veggie Power Base (2 Veggies)

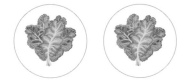

Add: 1 Fat + 2 Proteins + 1 Carb + 1 Fruit

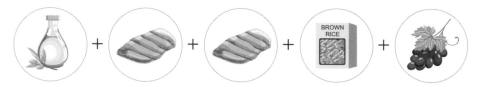

*You may substitute 2 Veggies for the 1 Fruit in this formula if desired.

Mean Bean

Start with: Vital Veggie Power Base (2 Veggies)

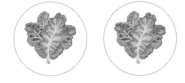

Add: 1 Fat + 2 Beans & Peas

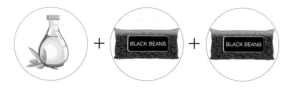

Note: To choose veggies, see page 155; carbs, page 158; fruits, page 161; proteins, page 163; fats, page 166; beans & peas, page 168; milks & yogurt, page 170.

Mix It Up

Start with: Vital Veggie Power Base (2 Veggies)

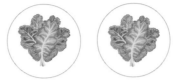

Add: 1 Fat + 1 Protein + 1 Beans & Peas + 1 Carb

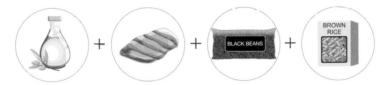

Supercharged Carb Power Meals

Remember that because, pound for pound, carbs have more calories than veggies, this Power Base will take up less space on your plate than the Vital Veggies do. You are going to start with one of the carbs from the list on page 158, add a fat, lots of veggies, and then some protein, beans, or milk, depending on your mood. You'll end up with a healthy, well-portioned meal that may include foods you've never imagined before: an open-faced sandwich on sprouted wheat bread; a blueberry yogurt parfait with muesli; or a veggie, tofu, and black bean stir-fry. The formula you choose from the list below depends on what protein you feel like eating (or happen to have in your kitchen!). Check out Chapter 11 for some examples of what these formulas look like.

Whole grains will naturally have more dietary fiber than the white stuff. You'll also be getting lots of extra fiber from the veggies, beans, peas, and legumes you'll be eating. As you increase the fiber in your diet, be sure to drink more water to keep your digestive system running smoothly—but you'll already be doing that anyway!

Pure Protein

Start with: Supercharged Carb Power Base (1 Carb)

Add: 1 Fat + 2 Proteins + 1 Veggie + 1 Fruit

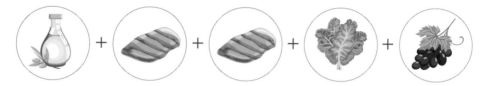

*You may substitute 2 Veggies for the 1 Fruit in this formula if desired.
*You may also substitute ½ Fruit for the 1 Veggie in this formula if desired.

Mean Bean

Start with: Supercharged Carb Power Base (1 Carb)

Add: 1 Fat = 1 protein + ½ Beans & Peas + 2 Veggies

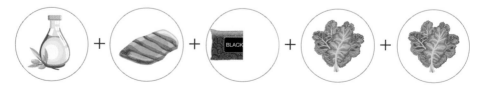

*You may substitute ½ Fruit for 1 of the 2 Veggies in this formula if desired.

Note: To choose veggies, see page 155; carbs, page 158; fruits, page 161; proteins, page 163; fats, page 166; beans & peas, page 168; milks & yogurt, page 170.

Dairy Does It

Start with: Supercharged Carb Power Base (1 Carb)

Add: 1 Fat + 1½ Milks & Yogurt + ½ Fruit

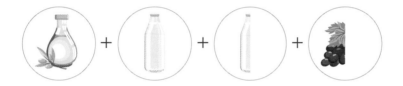

Power Drinks

Making your own yogurt-based fruit and veggie drinks at home is a quick and easy way to get more nutrition in! The Sugar Savvy Meal Plan calls for just one Power Drink a day, but if you're in a hurry, you can occasionally replace a Power Meal with a Power Drink. Note: BEWARE of store-bought smoothies. A lot of women will buy ready-made smoothies thinking they are saving time, but these are nothing but milk shakes in disguise. **Don't buy them! Instead, MAKE your own!**

There are a number of new machines out there to help you make these in a snap, but a good old-fashioned blender will do just fine. Always check your owner's manual to see how much preparation the fruits and veggies will need before you mix them up. Do you have to chop them? Remove the core? Remove the seeds of certain fruits and veggies? Or can you just throw everything in whole? One thing to make sure of is that you're not using a true "juicing" machine when building our Power Drinks. You will lose some nutrients that way, and these drinks are meant to be packed with nutrients!

To decide which formula to follow, simply first decide what type of drink you'd like to have. Do you regularly include Greek yogurt in your diet and love it? Greek Goddess might be for you! Do you avoid dairy but still need to be sure to get plenty of calcium in your day? Go with our Nondairy Delight. Just want a fresh and antioxidant-rich pick-me-up? Then the Fruit and Veggie Refresher it is!

> Experiment with different fruit and veggie combos. **The possibilities are endless!**

No matter what you start with to make your Power Drink, all formulas require a healthy fat. Avocado, chia seeds, flaxseed meal, hemp seeds, or cacao nibs work great! (Most of these ingredients are available in the organic or specialty food aisles in your grocery store. If you can't find them there, check your local food stores like Vitamin Shoppe or Whole Foods or large retailers like Target or Walmart.) Additionally, all the formulas include fruits and veggies in varying amounts to pack them full of major nutrition! Experiment with different fruit and veggie combos. The possibilities are endless here and you can really throw in whatever you've got around. Fruits and veggies on their way to being too ripe or wilted are great to throw in! Get the nutrition out of them instead of throwing them in the compost pile or down the garbage disposal!

In some cases, the formulas call for added protein. Things like tofu, cottage cheese, or protein powder can be put to use here. When choosing a protein powder, check the ingredients list to be sure that it does not contain added sugar! A couple brands I like are:

- Boku's Super Protein, vegan (available at bokusuperfood.com)
- Tera's Whey Organic Plain Whey Protein (available at teraswhey.com and at retail sites nationwide)

Check out Chapter 11 for some examples of drinks made with these formulas.

Greek Goddess

Start with: ½ cup fat-free plain Greek yogurt

Add: 2 Veggies + 1½ Fruits + 2 Fats

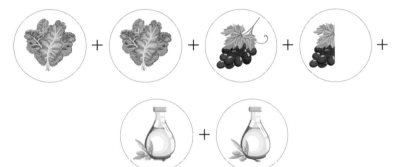

Nondairy Delight

Start with: 1 cup unsweetened soy milk or 2 cups unsweetened almond milk
(fortified with calcium and vitamins D and B12)

Add: 1 Veggie + 2 Fruits + 1 Protein + 1 Fat

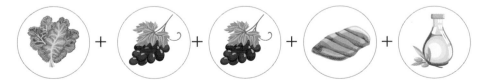

In the case of almond milk, choose one that has added protein.
In the case of soy milk, choose one that has been made from whole soy beans.

Note: To choose veggies, see page 155; carbs, page 158; fruits, page 161; proteins, page 163; fats, page 166; beans & peas, page 168; milks & yogurt, page 170.

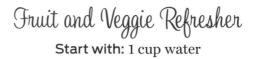

Fruit and Veggie Refresher

Start with: 1 cup water

Add: 2 Veggies + 2 Fruits + 2 Proteins + 1 Fat

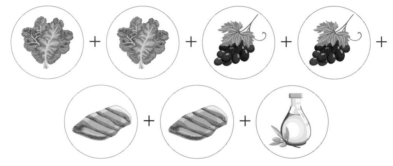

* You may increase or decrease the amount of water as desired.

PUTTING IT ALL TOGETHER

The guiding principle of Sugar Savvy eating is that everything you put in your mouth should help you get your ENERGY UP and your WEIGHT DOWN so you feel Fit, Fab, and Fierce all around! Here's what you are going to do on the Sugar Savvy Meal Plan:

❶ EAT (and sometimes DRINK) FOOD every 2 to 4 hours. You must fuel your body. I constantly hear people complaining that they don't eat all day and yet still can't lose weight. That's because you come home starving, so you eat anything and everything and your body puts it straight into storage because it's afraid you're going to starve it again. Plus, you can't possibly get all the nutrition you need every day if you're only eating in the evening. Focus on real foods that come from the earth. Your goal is to eliminate those that are processed.

2 **Eat or drink five Power Meals or Power Drinks each day.** Meals and drinks may be interchanged, combined, or split up depending on your needs and the constraints of your daily life, but I really *do* encourage you to eat regularly throughout the day. These mini-meals are lower in calories than the average American meal but they are loaded with fiber-rich foods, which will help you feel full and satisfied.

3 **Consume no more than 24 grams of added sugar in 24 hours.** Naturally occurring ones found in foods such as fruits and dairy products are fine. It's the added ones we're aiming to trash. This will be a snap if you follow the Sugar Savvy Meal Plan!

4 **Drink eight glasses of water a day.** I cannot say it enough . . . hydration is EXTREMELY important. Many times when you

For Emergencies: Energy Boosters!

Remember what I said before about always being prepared with Sugar Savvy foods? I know there are going to be days when you're stressed at work and need a little pick-me-up in the afternoon. I know there are going to be nights when you have a fight with your boyfriend that will send you straight to your fridge.

Ideally, you'll learn to find comfort in something other than food—call a friend or take a walk. But I also know that this is a process and during these six weeks of the plan especially, you may still turn to food. It's at these times that it's really critical that you reach for foods that will make you feel good, not foods that you'll hate yourself for eating later. It's at these times that our Energy Boosters can really come in handy. If you would normally go for something crunchy like chips, I'd suggest crunchy raw veggies or popcorn. If you feel like a doughnut or cookie, try a trail mix with some dried fruit or a fat-free latte.

These are lower in calories (and nutrition) than our Power Meals, so they can also be a great go-to when you're starting to get hungry, in a rush, or just need a little something before your next Power Meal. Try the following Energy Boosters when you're really stuck or really hungry:

* 2–3 cups of air-popped popcorn (sprinkle with nutritional yeast for a "cheesy" flavor and some protein)
* ¼–½ cup steamed edamame
* 8–12 oz fat-free caffe latte
* ¼–½ cup fresh fruit and one 1-oz low-fat string cheese
* Raw veggies and 2 Tbsp hummus
* A small handful of unsalted nuts or a trail mix with unsalted nuts and dried fruit (with no added sugar, of course)

THINK you are hungry, sleepy, depressed, or grouchy, you are really just dehydrated.

5 **Try to eat at least one High-Wattage Food per day.** Consult the list on page 170; these foods are also included in many Power Meal and Power Drink formulas. Many are high in free radical–fighting antioxidants, loaded with vitamins and minerals, and, in some cases, great sources of healthy fats. Have fun learning how to work these into your daily meal plan.

6 **Consider a daily whole food multivitamin with minerals.** It's best to get most of your nutrition from food—and the Sugar Savvy Meal Plan packs the nutrition in—but a multivitamin is a little added assurance that you are getting what you need each day. Choose a brand with no artificial preservatives, coloring, or flavors, and go organic if you can. I take New Chapter Every Woman Multivitamin. Solgar is another good brand. Talk to your healthcare provider about which one is best for you.

Some Things to Think About

As with any healthy eating plan, remember that one size does not fit all and that many foods, drinks, herbs, spices, and dietary supplements can interact with some medications. Especially if you are pregnant or nursing, or you have a chronic medical condition, please discuss the Sugar Savvy Meal Plan with your physician or healthcare provider first.

You should never feel deprived or starving on this plan. If you do, you may need a little more energy in the form of healthy foods. Calorie needs vary from person to person and really from day to day. The Sugar Savvy Meal Plan was designed to provide the appropriate nutrition and calorie level for women of average height and weight who are mostly sedentary and interested in losing weight. If you're tall or very active or don't have weight to lose, you may need to eat more. Try an Energy Booster or add an extra Power Meal or Drink.

It is important to eat a variety of food to ensure you are getting key nutrients. Don't fall into the trap of finding a few things you like and just eating the same things over and over. Variety helps fight food boredom, keeps your taste buds alive, sharpens your eating intuition, and ensures that you get all the nutrients you need. Varying the formulas you choose to build Power Meals and Power Drinks each day will help to ensure that you're doing this (and making your own swaps and substitutions will be second nature after a few weeks), but here are a few things to consider:

- Include at least 1 Beans & Peas serving in at least one meal a day.

- Include leafy greens in at least one meal a day (and try new ones all the time!).

- Include fish at least twice a week.

- To get adequate calcium and vitamin D daily, aim for 3 or more servings of high-calcium foods a day. You can find calcium in milk, cheeses, yogurt, and fortified nondairy beverages, of course, but also look to leafy greens (such as collards, kale, and turnip greens), nuts and seeds (such as almonds and sesame and chia seeds), soy beans, tofu, and more.

Feeling overwhelmed? Take a deep breath. I know this sounds like a lot to keep in mind—but I promise that it gets easier! Once you start shopping and cooking, you'll find that the formulas make it simple to eat Sugar Savvy.

The easiest place to start is with the sample week's menu you'll find in Week 2 of the Sugar Savvy plan (pages 102–103). If you're allergic to or just don't like something in this sample week, substitute a different food from the appropriate food group when making your meal—or swap out one of the meals entirely and instead try one of the 40 Power Meals or Drinks Jessica has provided for you in Chapter 11 (pages 191-215). When you're ready, start making your own Power Meals following the formulas and guidelines in this chapter.

SUGAR SAVVY
MEALS FOR LIFE

Power Meals and Power Drinks
to satisfy every taste bud!

"I really enjoy having all these creative formulas to choose from. It makes eating healthfully so interesting. I never get bored from always eating the same thing."

—MADELINE DE LA CRUZ, 22, ENERGY UP! ALUMNA
WHO LOST 55 POUNDS AFTER GETTING SUGAR SAVVY

Changing what you like is one thing. Knowing how to put all these new foods together in meals is another! Believe me, I understand! Here you will find 40 specific "recipes" for meals and drinks using the Power Meal formulas. They are designed to be a guide, so you develop a sense of how much of each Sugar Savvy food group to use and how to combine them for nourishing, satisfying, delicious results. Once you make a few of these amazing recipes, you'll have the know-how and confidence to put together your own wonderful creations!

Jessica has made these with her favorite brands to help narrow down your hunt through the grocery store, but you can use any nutritional equivalent. Just always remember to read your labels and watch out for added sugar and its evil sidekicks, excess salt, unhealthy fat, and enriched white flour!

When recipes call for roasting, use a nonfat cooking spray (preferably one that uses olive or coconut oil). Or purchase an atomized spraying device or mister, such as the Misto, Cuisipro Spray Pump, Cassia Oil Spray Pump, or RSVP Oil Mister. This handy kitchen tool can be found in most home and kitchen stores, department stores, and large retailers like Target or Walmart. Note that the minimal amount of oil used in this manner is not counted in the Power Meal formulas.

All of the recipes here make one Power Meal. But to make sure you are always PREPARED, you may want to make larger batches of each Power Meal; just multiply the ingredients as needed and adjust cooking times accordingly. Remember that you'll be enjoying five Power Meals or Drinks every day, every 2 to 4 hours.

BREAKFASTS

Cottage Cheese Medley

Supercharged Carb Power Base: Pure Protein

1 Carb + 1 Fat + 2 Proteins + ½ Fruit (substituted for 1 Veggie) + 1 Fruit

1 slice toasted sprouted whole grain bread + 1 Tbsp flaxseed meal &
2 chopped walnut halves + ½ cup low-fat, no-sodium-added cottage
cheese + ½ peach, sliced + ¾ cup mango cubes + seasonings (cinnamon
and/or cardamom)

Combine the cottage cheese and flaxseed meal. Top the toasted bread with
the cottage cheese mixture, sliced fruit, and walnuts. Sprinkle with cinnamon
and/or cardamom to taste.

Homemade Granola with Greek Yogurt

Supercharged Carb Power Base: Dairy Does It

1 Carb + 1 Fat + 1½ Milks & Yogurt + ½ Fruit

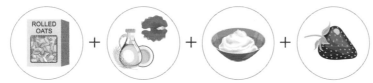

¼ cup dry old-fashioned rolled oats + ½ tsp melted
coconut oil & 2 chopped walnut halves + 9 oz fat-free
plain Greek yogurt + ½ cup sliced or whole strawberries

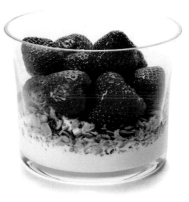

Preheat the oven to 300ºF. Combine the oats and
walnuts with the melted coconut oil and place on a baking
sheet. Bake until the oats are lightly browned (about 5 to
10 minutes). Remove from the oven and let cool. Top the
Greek yogurt with the oat mixture and fruit.

*Note that the ¼ cup dry rolled oats will roughly double to ½ cup in
cooking.*

Yogurt Parfait

Supercharged Carb Power Base: Dairy Does It
1 Carb + 1 Fat + 1½ Milks & Yogurt + ½ Fruit

¼ cup no-added-sugar Swiss muesli + 2 Tbsp flaxseed meal + 9 oz fat-free plain yogurt + ½ cup fresh blackberries

Place yogurt in the bottom of a parfait cup. Top with alternating layers of all additional ingredients.

Hot Breakfast Cereal with Cranberries and Walnuts

Supercharged Carb Power Base: Dairy Does It
1 Carb + 1 Fat + 1½ Milks & Yogurt + ½ Fruit

½ cup prepared Bob's Red Mill 8-Grain Hot Cereal + 4 chopped walnut halves + 1½ cups skim milk + 1½ tablespoons unsweetened dried cranberries

Prepare the cereal with ¾ cup skim milk instead of water. (Omit salt, if called for.) Top with the walnuts and cherries and serve the remaining ¾ cup skim milk on the side.

Oatmeal with Almonds and Blueberries

Supercharged Carb Power Base: Dairy Does It
1 Carb + 1 Fat + 1½ Milks & Yogurt + ½ Fruit

½ cup prepared steel-cut oats + 8 sliced or chopped almonds + 1½ cups unsweetened almond milk + ½ cup blueberries + seasoning (cinnamon)

Prepare the oats according to instructions, using the unsweetened almond milk. (Omit salt, if called for.) Top with the blueberries, almonds, and cinnamon.

To save time in the morning, start your oatmeal the night before, or make a big batch in the beginning of the week and reheat some in the microwave as needed. Note that 1 cup dry steel-cut oats + 4 cups liquid = 6 (½ cup) servings of oatmeal. You can also trade the blueberries for raisins or unsweetened applesauce!

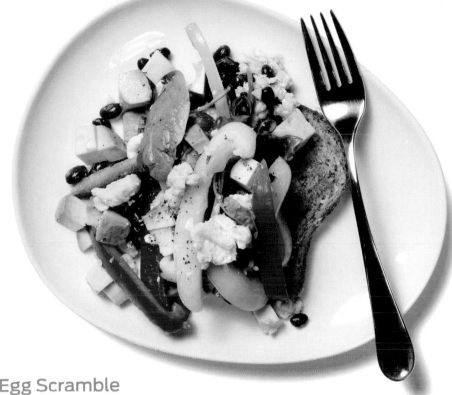

Avocado Egg Scramble

Vital Veggie Power Base: Mix It Up
2 Veggies + 1 Fat + 1 Protein + 1 Beans & Peas + 1 Carb

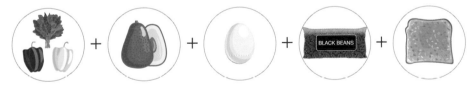

1 cup baby spinach & ½ cup sliced red bell pepper & ½ cup sliced yellow bell pepper + 2 Tbsp chopped avocado + 1 large egg, beaten + ½ cup cooked black beans + 1 slice sprouted wheat toast + seasonings (red pepper flakes & 1 clove minced garlic)

Spray a sauté pan with nonfat cooking spray (preferably using olive or coconut oil). Sauté the thinly sliced red and yellow bell peppers with the garlic and red pepper flakes. Add the egg and scramble until firm. Add the black beans and warm through. Add the spinach and cook until just wilted. Serve with the avocado and 1 slice sprouted wheat bread.

Eggs and "Hash Browns"

Supercharged Carb Power Base: Pure Protein

1 Carb + 1 Fat + 2 Proteins + 1 Veggie + 1 Fruit

½ cup cubed red potatoes + 1 tsp coconut oil + 1 oz low-sodium, low-fat cheese (such as cheddar or Colby) & 1 egg + ¾ cup baby spinach & ¼ cup sun-dried tomatoes + 1 cup sliced strawberries + seasoning (chopped fresh rosemary)

Preheat the oven to 350°F. Use a sprayer to mist the potatoes with olive oil, sprinkle them with the fresh chopped rosemary, and roast them in a rimmed baking sheet for about 15 to 20 minutes, or until slightly browned. In the meantime, melt the coconut oil in a sauté pan. Add the spinach and sun-dried tomatoes and cook until the spinach is slightly wilted. Scramble the egg and pour it into the sauté pan over the spinach. Cook until the egg is firm. Add the cheese, and cook until melted. Plate the eggs with the potatoes and garnish with the strawberries.

Eggs over Greens and Grains

Vital Veggie Power Base: Pure Protein

2 Veggies + 1 Fat + 2 Proteins + 1 Carb + 1 Fruit

1½ cups arugula & ½ cup diced shallots + 1 tsp coconut oil + 2 eggs, poached or fried using nonfat cooking spray + ½ cup cooked brown rice + 1 cup orange segments + seasoning (1 clove minced garlic)

Sauté the diced shallots and garlic in the coconut oil. Add the arugula and heat until wilted through. Transfer to a plate, top with the eggs, and serve with the brown rice and orange segments.

SALADS

Southwest Steak Salad

Vital Veggie Power Base: Mix It Up

2 Veggies + 1 Fat + 1 Protein + 1 Beans & Peas + 1 Carb

1 cup chopped kale & ½ cup chopped plum tomatoes or grape tomatoes & ¼ cup thinly sliced red bell peppers & ¼ cup thinly sliced jicama + 2 Tbsp chopped avocado + 1 oz grilled flank steak + ½ cup cooked black beans + ½ cup cooked corn + seasoning (lemon or lime juice)

Wash the kale and separate the ribs from the leaves. Discard the ribs and chop the leaves. Top with the remaining ingredients and dress with a little olive oil and a squeeze of lemon or lime juice.

Tossing this salad a little ahead of time can help to soften the kale leaves. If you don't have jicama on hand, just have more of the other veggies! Add chopped cilantro, if desired. You can also substitute grilled chicken for the flank steak, if desired.

Barley, Artichoke, and Chicken Salad

Supercharged Carb Power Base: Pure Protein

1 Carb + 1 Fat + 2 Proteins + 1 Veggie + 1 Fruit

½ cup cooked barley + 1 tsp olive oil + 2 oz shredded grilled chicken + ½ cup quartered artichokes & ¼ cup diced red onion & ¼ cup grape tomatoes, cut in half + 1 cup pear slices + seasoning (red wine vinegar & chopped parsley)

Combine the first 6 ingredients. Drizzle with a little red wine vinegar and chopped parsley. Serve with the sliced pears on the side.

Add 2 cups of additional veggies instead of the fruit, if desired. You can simply increase the amount of the veggies used in the recipe or serve the salad as is with a side of leafy greens. You can also substitute grilled salmon or feta cheese for the chicken, if desired. You can also substitute wheat berries or farro for the barley. Note that some brands or varieties of wheat berries may require soaking overnight.

Sweet Potato Salad

Vital Veggie Power Base: Pure Protein

2 Veggies + 1 Fat + 2 Proteins + 1 Carb + 2 Veggies (substituted in for 1 Fruit)

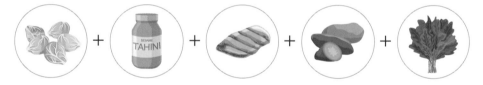

2 cups Brussels sprouts, trimmed and halved + 2 tsp tahini + 2 oz grilled chicken breast + ½ cup peeled and cubed sweet potatoes + 2 cups baby spinach

Preheat the oven to 350°F. Mix the Brussels sprouts with the sweet potatoes and mist them with olive oil. Roast for about 20 to 30 minutes, or until the vegetables are tender. Mix the warm vegetables with the spinach and tahini. Serve with a side of grilled chicken breast.

You can also try this meal with pork tenderloin or grilled salmon instead of chicken. If it's more convenient, roast the Brussels sprouts and sweet potatoes ahead of time and serve them cold OR warm them up in the microwave!

Crunchy Tuna Salad

Vital Veggie Power Base: Pure Protein

2 Veggies + 1 Fat + 2 Proteins + 1 Carb + 1 Fruit

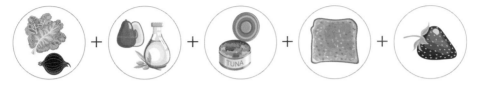

1½ cups chopped kale (ribs removed and discarded) & ½ cup diced red onion + ½ tsp olive oil & 1 Tbsp diced avocado + 2 oz tuna canned in water (drained) + 1 piece sprouted wheat bread + 1 cup sliced strawberries

Toast the wheat bread and cut it into cubes to make homemade croutons. Mix the tuna with the chopped red onion and olive oil. Serve atop a bed of the kale, avocado, sliced berries, and croutons.

Use about half of a 5-oz can of tuna and save the rest for another meal. Sub extra veggies for the strawberries for a more savory salad. Leftover artichokes, additional red onion, and grape tomatoes would work great here. Olives can be used in place of the avocado. And you can use any leafy greens in place of the kale; try mesclun or spring greens.

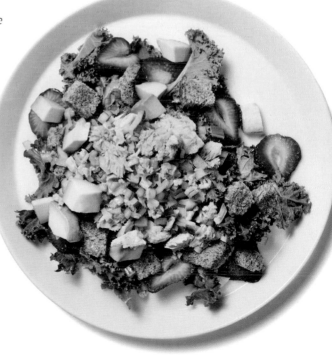

Simple Salmon Salad

Vital Veggies Power Base: Pure Protein

2 Veggies + 1 Fat + 2 Proteins + 1 Carb + 2 Veggies (substituted in for 1 Fruit)

1 cup baby spinach and 1 cup baby kale (ribs removed and discarded) + 1 tsp olive oil + 2 oz grilled salmon + ½ cup cooked corn & ¾ cup grape tomatoes & ¼ cup chopped red onion + seasoning (red wine vinegar)

Wash and prepare the spinach and kale. Combine with the remaining ingredients. Dress with a little red wine vinegar.

You can try grilled shrimp or chicken for a great twist on this salad. Freshly husked corn off the cob is a special treat, but when you're in a hurry, go with frozen yellow corn.

"Grilled" Veggie Salad

Vital Veggie Power Base: Mean Bean

2 Veggies + 1 Fat + 2 Beans & Peas

¾ cup spring greens and spinach & ¼ cup sliced mushrooms & 3 spears steamed asparagus & ¼ cup sliced red bell peppers & ¼ cup julienned sun-dried tomatoes + 1 tsp olive oil + ½ cup cooked black beans & ½ cup cooked kidney beans + seasoning (balsamic vinegar or Bragg's Liquid Aminos)

Sauté the sliced mushrooms, sliced red bell peppers, and sun-dried tomatoes in ¼ tsp of the olive oil until tender. Add the steamed asparagus and beans and heat until warmed through. Plate the greens and top with the warm sautéed vegetables. Dress with the remaining olive oil and a little balsamic vinegar or Bragg's liquid aminos to taste.

You may use any combination of vegetables to top the salad. If you have a grill available, you can actually grill the veggies in a grill basket or wrapped in aluminum foil. Drizzle with a little olive oil, add any additional dried herbs or spices you'd like, wrap, and grill!

Broccoli and Chickpea Salad

Vital Veggie Power Base: Mean Bean

2 Veggies + 1 Fat + 2 Beans & Peas

1 cup chopped broccoli & 1 cup finely chopped arugula + 1 tsp olive oil +
1 cup cooked chickpeas + seasoning (½ tsp Dijon mustard)

To prepare the dressing: In a small bowl, whisk together the Dijon mustard and olive oil. You may add additional herbs, such as finely chopped chives, if you want.

For the salad: Combine the broccoli, arugula, and chickpeas in a large bowl. Toss with the prepared dressing.

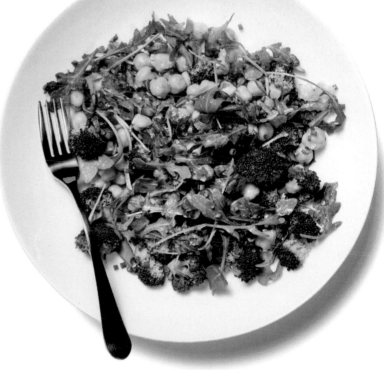

Caprese Salad

Vital Veggie Power Base: Pure Protein

2 Veggies + 1 Fat + 2 Proteins + 1 Carb + 1 Fruit

1 cup diced tomatoes & ¼ cup diced red onion & ¾ cup chopped spinach + 1 tsp olive oil + 2 oz diced part-skim mozzarella cheese + 1 slice sprouted whole wheat bread or 13 Mary's Gone Crackers + 1 cup Granny Smith apple slices + seasoning (red wine vinegar or balsamic vinegar)

Mix the tomatoes, red onion, spinach, olive oil, and cheese together and add red wine vinegar or balsamic vinegar, to taste. Serve with the bread or crackers and apple slices on the side.

Avocado and Cottage Cheese Dippers

Vital Veggie Power Base: Pure Protein

2 Veggies + 1 Fat + 2 Proteins + 1 Carb + 1 Fruit

½ cup thinly sliced red bell peppers & 1 cup thinly sliced zucchini & ½ cup thinly sliced carrots + 2 Tbsp avocado, mashed + ½ cup low-fat, no-sodium-added cottage cheese + 13 Mary's Gone Crackers + 1 banana (about 6" long) + seasoning (1 clove minced garlic)

Mix the cottage cheese with the avocado and minced garlic until well blended. Use the avocado and cottage cheese mixture as a dip for the julienned vegetables and as a spread for the crackers. Enjoy the banana on the side.

For a smoother texture, blend the dip ingredients in a blender. Vary your veggies each time you have this easy Power Meal. Try jicama, okra, cucumber, or celery. You can also change up the fruit each time!

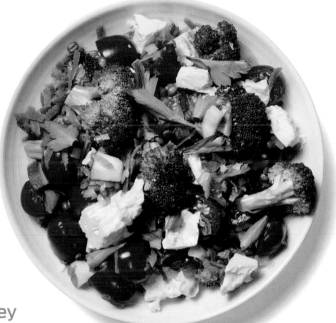

Warm Vegetable Medley

Supercharged Carb: Pure Protein

1 Carb + 1 Fat + 2 Proteins + 1 Veggie + 2 Veggies (substituted for 1 Fruit)

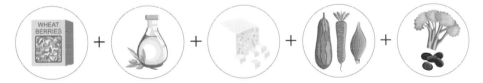

½ cup cooked wheat berries + 1 tsp olive oil + 2 oz fat-free or reduced-fat feta cheese + ½ cup shredded carrots & ¼ cup diced zucchini & ¼ cup minced shallots + 1 cup chopped broccoli & 1 cup halved grape tomatoes + seasonings (red wine vinegar & chopped parsley)

Sauté the broccoli, shredded carrots, grape tomatoes, zucchini, and shallots in the olive oil. Combine the veggies with the prepared wheat berries and top with the feta cheese. Drizzle with red wine vinegar and chopped parsley.

Substitute grilled chicken for the feta cheese if you'd like.

SANDWICHES

Chicken Enchiladas

Vital Veggie Power Base: Mix It Up

2 Veggies + 1 Fat + 1 Protein + 1 Beans & Peas + 1 Carb

¼ cup thinly sliced green pepper & ¼ cup thinly sliced yellow onion & ½ cup chopped plum tomatoes or grape tomatoes + ½ tsp olive oil & 1 Tbsp chopped avocado + 1 oz grilled chicken + ½ cup cooked black beans + 1–2 sprouted corn tortillas + seasonings (low-sodium chicken broth & cumin or chipotle chili powder)

Sauté the peppers and onions in the olive oil. Add the chicken and black beans once the veggies are slightly softened. Add low-sodium chicken broth or water as needed to keep the chicken from drying out, along with cumin or chipotle chili powder. Wrap it all in the warmed corn tortillas. Top with the chopped tomatoes and avocado.

Open-Faced Tuna Salad Sandwich

Supercharged Carb Power Base: Pure Protein

1 Carb + 1 Fat + 2 Proteins + 1 Veggie + 1 Fruit

1 slice sprouted whole grain bread, toasted + 1 tsp olive oil + 2 oz tuna canned in water + ¼ cup quartered artichokes & ¼ cup diced red onion & ¼ cup grape tomatoes, finely chopped or diced & ¼ cup fresh spinach leaves + 1 serving red grapes (about 17)

Drain the tuna and combine it with the olive oil, red onion, artichokes, and tomatoes. Place the spinach leaves atop the toasted bread and finish with the tuna salad. Serve with a side of grapes or fruit of your choosing.

Open-Faced "Egg Salad" Sandwich

Supercharged Carb Power Base: Pure Protein

1 Carb + 1 Fat + 2 Proteins + 1 Veggie + 1 Fruit

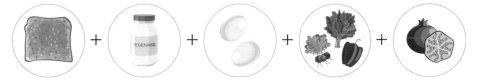

1 slice sprouted whole grain bread, toasted + 2 tsp Vegenaise + 2 hard-boiled eggs + ½ cup baby spinach leaves & ¼ cup thinly sliced radishes & ¼ cup julienned red bell peppers + ½ cup pomegranate arils or seeds

Spread the Vegenaise over the toasted bread. Top with the spinach leaves, radishes, and peppers. Slice the hard-boiled eggs and add them to the sandwich. Serve with the arils (seeds) from the pomegranate. (If you don't like them on the sandwich, enjoy the pomegranate seeds on the side).

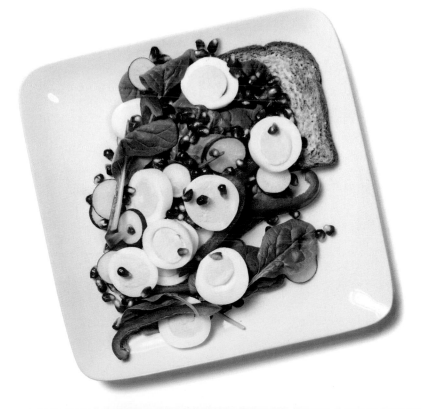

Sweet Summer Salad and Sandwich Combo

Vital Veggie Power Base: Pure Protein

2 Veggies + 1 Fat + 2 Proteins + 1 Carb + 1 Fruit

1½ cups chopped arugula & ½ cup thinly sliced shallots + ½ tsp extra virgin olive oil + 1 Tbsp avocado, mashed + 2 oz sliced low-fat cheese + 1 slice sprouted whole wheat bread + 1 fresh fig, sliced & ½ cup sliced strawberries + seasonings (½–1 tsp champagne vinegar & ½ clove minced garlic)

For the sandwich: Toast the bread and cut it in half. Spread one half with the avocado and layer with the cheese and the other half of the bread.

For the salad: Combine the champagne vinegar with the garlic. Add the olive oil and whisk to complete the vinaigrette. Combine the chopped arugula with the shallots and dress with the prepared vinaigrette. Slice the strawberries and fig and scatter them on top.

Cheesy Avocado-Tomato Topped English Muffin

Vital Veggie Power Base: Mix It Up

2 Veggies + 1 Fat + 1 Protein + 1 Beans & Peas + 1 Carb

1 cup mesclun & ½ cup roasted tomatoes & ½ cup sliced cucumber + ½ tsp olive oil & 1 Tbsp sliced avocado + 1 slice (1 oz) reduced-fat Swiss cheese + ½ cup cooked chickpeas + ½ sprouted whole grain English muffin, toasted + seasonings (balsamic, red wine, or apple cider vinegar & fresh basil leaves)

Place the cheese on the English muffin. Top with the fresh basil leaves, roasted tomatoes, and sliced avocado. Serve with a side salad made with the mesclun, cucumbers, and chickpeas. Dress the salad with the olive oil and vinegar of your choosing. Try balsamic, red wine, or apple cider vinegar.

Change up this dish by using sun-dried tomatoes or roasted red peppers in place of the roasted tomatoes.

Portobello Cheese Steak

Supercharged Carb Power Base: Mean Bean

1 Carb + 1 Fat + 1 Protein + ½ Beans & Peas + 2 Veggies

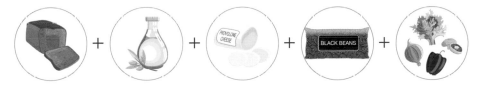

1 slice sprouted whole grain bread, toasted + 1 tsp olive oil + 1 slice (1 oz) low-fat provolone + ¼ cup black beans, cooked and mashed with a fork or pureed into a paste + 1 medium (4 oz) portobello mushroom, sliced & ¼ cup diced or sliced yellow onion & ¼ cup roasted red peppers & ½ cup spring greens

Preheat the broiler. Sauté the mushrooms, onions, and peppers in the olive oil until softened. Top the toasted bread with the greens, mashed black beans, sautéed veggies, and cheese. Place on a broiling pan and broil until the cheese has melted.

Roasted Eggplant and Tomato Sandwich

Supercharged Carb Power Base: Mean Bean

1 Carb + 1 Fat + 1 Protein + ½ Beans & Peas + 2 Veggies

½ sprouted whole grain English muffin, toasted + 1 tsp olive oil + 1 slice (1 oz) low-fat goat cheese + ¼ cup cooked chickpeas + 1 thick slice eggplant & 1 thick slice tomato & 1½ cups Swiss chard + seasoning (red wine or balsamic vinegar)

Combine ¾ tsp of the olive oil and the beans in a food processor or blender and puree. Mist the eggplant and tomato slices with olive oil and roast them in a 350ºF oven for about 10 to 15 minutes (turning once), until tender. Top the toasted English muffin with the pureed garbanzo beans, a few of the leafy greens, the roasted tomato and eggplant slices, and finally, the cheese slice. Place back in the oven and broil on high heat until the cheese is melted.

Serve with a side of Swiss chard. You may dress it with the remaining olive oil and red wine or balsamic vinegar or sauté it in the remaining olive oil.

ENTREES

Grilled Chicken Salsa

Vital Veggie Power Base: Mix It Up

2 Veggies + 1 Fat + 1 Protein + 1 Beans & Peas + 1 Carb

1½ cups cherry tomatoes, cut in half & ¼ cup diced green onion & ¼ cup diced red onion + 1 tsp olive oil + 1 oz diced or shredded grilled chicken + ½ cup cooked black beans + ½ cup cooked corn + seasonings (cumin, chili powder, ground black pepper, red wine vinegar & if desired, cilantro)

Season the chicken with cumin and chili powder, and heat it through in a sauté pan. Mix the chicken with vegetables, beans, and corn, and season with ground black pepper and red wine vinegar. You can also add cilantro for a little zing.

This can easily be made with tofu instead of chicken. Get extra-firm light tofu and use about 1 to 3 ounces.

Veggie Chili

Vital Veggie Power Base: Mix It Up

2 Veggies + 1 Fat + 1 Protein + 1 Beans & Peas + 1 Carb

1 cup diced tomatoes & ½ cup chopped green bell peppers & ¼ cup chopped onion & ¼ cup diced zucchini & finely chopped spinach or collard greens (optional) + 1 tsp olive oil + 1 oz shredded low-fat cheese + ½ cup cooked kidney beans + ½ cup cooked corn + seasoning (chili powder, see box below & if desired, low-sodium vegetable broth)

Sauté the peppers, onion, and zucchini in the olive oil until the onions start to become translucent. Then stir in the diced tomatoes, beans, greens (if using), and corn. Add the desired amount of chili seasoning and bring to a boil. You may add additional liquid if needed at this point. Use water or low-sodium vegetable broth. Reduce the heat to low and simmer for about 20 minutes. Top with cheese and enjoy!

Make Your Own Chili Seasoning

Beware! Most commercial chili seasonings are loaded with flour, salt, and sugar. So make your own ahead of time, or just toss in the individual spices below as you're cooking.

* ¼ cup quinoa, spelt, or buckwheat flour
* 2 tsp chili powder
* 1 Tbsp dried minced onion
* 1 Tbsp dried minced garlic
* 1 tsp coconut palm sugar
* 2 tsp ground cumin
* 2 tsp dried parsley
* 2 tsp salt
* 1 tsp dried basil
* ¼ tsp ground black pepper

Sugar Savvy Nachos

Supercharged Carb Power Base: Mean Bean

1 Carb + 1 Fat + 1 Protein + ½ Beans & Peas + 2 Veggies

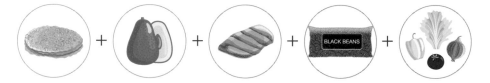

1–2 sprouted whole grain corn tortillas + 2 Tbsp chopped avocado + 1 oz shredded grilled chicken + ¼ cup cooked black beans + 2 cups chopped firm veggies such as bell peppers, tomatoes, lettuce & red onion + seasonings (cumin, chili powder, garlic powder & if desired, Bragg's Liquid Aminos & chopped cilantro)

Preheat the oven to 350°F. Lightly spray each tortilla with olive oil, then cut them into quarters. (You can cut them smaller if you'd like "more," but bigger is better for scooping.) Arrange in a single layer on a baking sheet and bake for 8 to 12 minutes. (Check halfway, as you may need to rotate your pan.) In the meantime, spray a nonstick skillet with a tiny amount of extra virgin olive oil. Sauté some of the chopped veggies until slightly tender. Add the chicken, black beans, cumin, chili powder, and garlic powder, and cook until heated through. Remove the tortilla chips from the oven and top them with the sautéed veggie mixture, additional chopped veggies, and chopped avocado. You can also add a few drops of Bragg's Liquid Aminos and chopped cilantro for a perfect finish!

Thanksgiving Dinner

Supercharged Carb Power Base: Mean Bean

1 Carb + 1 Fat + 1 Protein + ½ Beans & Peas + 1 Veggie + ½ Fruit (substituted for 1 Veggie)

½ cup sweet potato + 1 tsp coconut oil + 1 oz roasted turkey breast + ¼ cup cooked white cannellini beans + 1 cup green beans, steamed & ½ cup peeled, sliced apples + seasonings (minced garlic, grated fresh ginger & cumin)

Prick holes in the sweet potato and microwave it on high power for 5 to 8 minutes (until soft). Remove ½ cup of potato from the skin and save the rest for another Power Meal. In the meantime, melt 1 tsp coconut oil in a small sauté pan. Add a dash of the garlic, ginger, and cumin and cook for 30 seconds. Add the diced apple and cook until softened. Add the cannellini beans and heat through. Place the bean and apple mixture in a food processor or blender. Add the sweet potatoes and blend until smooth. Serve with the roasted turkey breast and green beans.

Beans 'n' Greens Pasta

Supercharged Carb Power Base: Mean Bean

1 Carb + 1 Fat + 1 Protein + ½ Beans & Peas + 2 Veggies

½ cup cooked sprouted whole grain pasta + 1 tsp extra virgin olive oil + 1 oz nonfat grated Parmesan cheese + ¼ cup cooked dark red kidney beans + 1 cup kale & ½ cup Swiss chard or collard greens & ½ cup grape tomatoes + seasonings (1 tsp minced garlic & if desired, 1–2 Tbsp low-sodium chicken or vegetable broth & cooked shallots and/or onions)

Heat the olive oil in a sauté pan on medium-high heat. Add the minced garlic and sauté for 1 minute. Add the grape tomatoes and cook until soft. Add the kidney beans and heat through. Remove the pan from the heat, add the greens, and cover until wilted. (You may also add chicken or vegetable broth at this time if more liquid is desired.) Add the beans and greens mixture to the ⅓ cup cooked pasta, top with grated Parmesan, and enjoy. You may also add cooked shallots and/or onions, if desired.

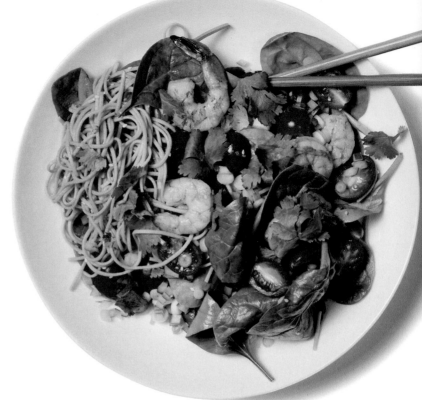

Sesame Noodles with Shrimp

Supercharged Carb: Pure Protein

1 Carb + 1 Fat + 2 Proteins + 1 Veggie + 2 Veggies (substituted for
1 Fruit)

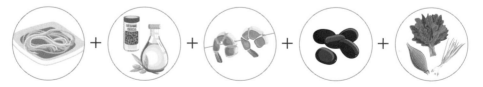

¾ cup cooked soba or buckwheat noodles + ⅔ tsp coconut oil & 1 tsp
sesame seeds + 2 oz grilled shrimp + 1 cup halved grape tomatoes +
1½ cups baby spinach leaves & ¼ cup chopped green onions & ¼ cup
finely chopped shallots or red onion + seasonings (rice wine vinegar &
if desired, cilantro)

Combine all of the above ingredients. Add rice wine vinegar to taste and top
with chopped fresh cilantro, if desired. May serve chilled or warm.

Better Butternut Squash

Supercharged Carb Power Base: Mean Bean

1 Carb + 1 Fat + 1 Protein + ½ Beans & Peas + 2 Veggies

½ cup roasted butternut squash, cut into cubes + 1 Tbsp diced avocado & ½ tsp olive oil + ¼ cup low-fat no-added-sodium cottage cheese + ¼ cup cooked lentils + 1½ cups chopped kale (ribs removed and discarded) & ½ cup roasted beets

Sauté the kale in the olive oil. Top the roasted butternut squash with the sautéed kale, cooked lentils, avocado, roasted beets, and cottage cheese.

Try Swiss chard or collard greens instead of the kale, or go for a mix of all three!

Spaghetti Squash with Roasted Red Peppers

Supercharged Carb Power Base: Pure Protein

1 Carb + 1 Fat + 2 Proteins + 1 Veggie + 2 Veggies (substituted for 1 Fruit)

1½ cups cooked spaghetti squash + 1 Tbsp reduced-fat cream cheese + 2 oz roasted chicken breast + 1 cup roasted red peppers + 2 cups baby spinach + seasonings (pinch ground red pepper & ¼ tsp red wine vinegar & ⅛ tsp roasted garlic paste)

Prick the squash all over and microwave it, turning occasionally, until tender to the touch, 12 to 15 minutes. Let cool for about 10 minutes. Cut the squash in half lengthwise and scoop out the seeds. Using a fork, scrape the squash into a bowl and separate it into strands. Use 1½ cups for this recipe and reserve the rest for another Power Meal!

Meanwhile, combine the roasted red peppers, vinegar, garlic paste, and ground red pepper in a food processor. Puree until smooth, about 2 minutes. Add the cream cheese and puree until incorporated, about 30 seconds. Steam the baby spinach in a vegetable steamer on the stovetop until just wilted. Combine the squash with the red pepper sauce and spinach. Serve with the roasted chicken breast.

Veggie Stir-Fry

Vital Veggie Power Base: Pure Protein

2 Veggies + 1 Fat + 2 Proteins + 1 Carb + 2 Veggies (substituted for 1 Fruit)

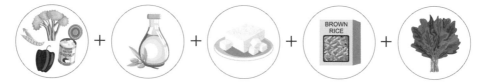

½ cup chopped red bell pepper & ½ cup water chestnuts & ½ cup broccoli & ½ cup snow peas + 1 tsp olive oil or coconut oil + 3–6 oz light tofu fortified with calcium and vitamins D and B12 (or the amount that contains ~14 grams of protein) + ½ cup cooked brown rice + 2 cups baby spinach + seasoning (1–2 cloves minced garlic)

Sauté the minced garlic, red bell pepper, water chestnuts, broccoli, and snow peas in the oil until tender. Add the tofu and heat through, followed by the baby spinach. Cook until the spinach is just wilted. Add the cooked brown rice and stir to combine all ingredients.

Swap in chicken instead of tofu, if you choose. To cut down on unused or leftover veggies, simply use up what you have in the fridge, as just about any combination can work in a stir-fry. Experiment with additional spices, too!

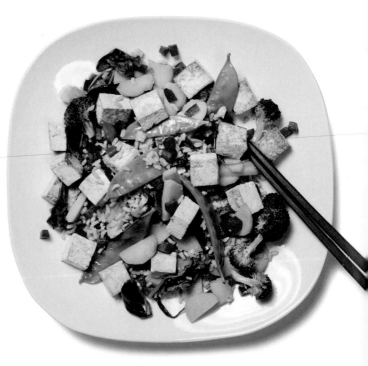

POWER DRINKS

Kale-Apple-Pear Power Drink

Greek Goddess

½ cup fat-free plain Greek yogurt + 2 Veggies + 1½ Fruits + 2 Fats

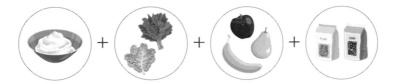

½ cup fat-free plain Greek yogurt + 1 cup chopped kale, ribs removed and discarded & 1 cup baby spinach + ½ cup sliced apple & ½ cup sliced pear & ½ small sliced banana + 2 Tbsp flaxseed meal & 1 Tbsp chia seeds

Combine all of the ingredients in a food processor or blender. Puree until smooth.

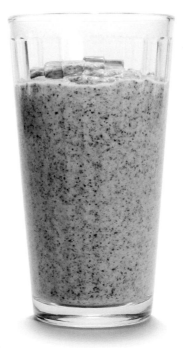

Cucumber-Grape Power Drink

Fruit and Veggie Refresher

1 cup water + 2 Veggies + 2 Fruits + 2 Proteins + 1 Fat

1 cup water + 1 cup chopped cucumber & 1 cup spinach & 17 red grapes & ¾ cup pineapple cubes + 3–6 oz light tofu fortified with calcium and vitamins D and B12 (or the amount that contains ~14 grams of protein) + 2 Tbsp chopped avocado

Combine all of the ingredients in a food processor or blender. Puree until smooth.

You may increase or decrease the amount of water as desired.

Spinach-Orange-Banana Power Drink

Greek Goddess

½ cup fat-free plain Greek yogurt + 2 Veggies + 1½ Fruits + 2 Fats

½ cup fat-free plain Greek yogurt + 2 cups spinach + 1 cup peeled orange segments & ½ banana + 2 Tbsp flaxseed meal & 1 Tbsp chia seeds

Combine all of the ingredients in a food processor or blender. Puree until smooth.

Kale-Mango Power Drink

Nondairy Delight

1 cup unsweetened soy milk (fortified with calcium and vitamins D and B12) + 1 Veggie + 2 Fruits + 1 Protein + 1 Fat

1 cup unsweetened soy milk + ½ cup chopped kale (ribs removed and discarded) & ½ cup chopped Swiss chard leaves + ¾ cup mango cubes & ¾ cup pineapple chunks + 1–3 oz light tofu fortified with calcium and vitamins D and B12 (or the amount that contains ~7 grams of protein) + 1 Tbsp chia seeds

Combine all of the ingredients in a food processor or blender. Puree until smooth.

Almond-Orange-Pineapple Power Drink

Nondairy Delight

2 cups unsweetened almond milk (fortified with calcium, vitamins D and B12, and added protein) + 1 Veggie + 2 Fruits + 1 Protein + 1 Fat

2 cups unsweetened almond milk + 1 cup spinach + 1 cup peeled orange segments & ¾ cup pineapple chunks + 1–3 oz light tofu fortified with calcium and vitamins D and B12 (or the amount that contains ~7 grams of protein) + 1 Tbsp chia seeds

Combine all of the ingredients in a food processor or blender. Puree until smooth.

You can use any greens in place of the spinach, if you'd like; sub in kale for extra calcium or use up greens that are on their way out!

Carrot-Berry Power Drink

Fruit and Veggie Refresher

1 cup water + 2 Veggies + 2 Fruits + 2 Proteins + 1 Fat

1 cup water + 1 cup chopped carrots & 1 cup baby spinach + 1 cup blueberries & 1 cup sliced strawberries + 3–6 oz light tofu fortified with calcium and vitamins D and B12 (or the amount that contains ~14 grams of protein) + 2 Tbsp chopped avocado

Combine all of the ingredients in a food processor or blender. Puree until smooth.

You may increase or decrease the amount of water as desired.

CHAPTER 12

THE SUGAR SAVVY WORKOUT

Moves to make you look as Fit, Fab, and Fierce as you feel!

"The Sugar Savvy plan is the only thing that makes me move. Because I am not someone who tends to be physically active. But I know it's important and I feel more creative and energetic since I've started moving more every day."

—ARLENE PINEDA, 58 ,
WHO LOST **9.4 POUNDS** IN **6 WEEKS**

Our bodies were designed to MOVE! Moving your body burns fat, strengthens your muscles, and gets your heart pumping so you get fresh oxygen and nutrient-rich blood coursing through your veins! Just as you feel sluggish and tired when you do nothing but sit, sit, sit, you will feel supercharged and energetic when you move, move, move! Energy is like a muscle. If you don't use it, you lose it!

> It's important to really believe in yourself and your ability to **kick sugar and self-doubt out** of your life for good.

I personally try to **move constantly.** I try to see how many squats I can do while I'm putting together dinner. I do arm curls while I watch TV. I stretch while I'm lying in bed. And my body thanks me for it by being fit, healthy, and pain free! I challenge you to do the same! Don't sit still when you can be on the move. Even if you're stuck at your desk, you can stand and stretch. Look for every opportunity to walk, run, ride a bike, dance, and move that body!

To help, I've created the Sugar Savvy Workout. Once you see how great it feels to move and shout and strengthen your muscles, you'll be hooked! There are two parts to the Sugar Savvy Workout: the Moving Affirmations and the Power Workout.

THE SUGAR SAVVY MOVING AFFIRMATIONS

As I described in Chapter 6, the Sugar Savvy Moving Affirmations are one of the most powerful weapons in your fight to retrain your brain. When you move your body the way it was designed to move, your brain releases endorphins that make you feel amazing. Shout out your affirmations as you do this, and your brain will automatically start to translate these positive thoughts into reality.

Do at least two Moving Affirmation series each day, starting with a warm-up and Energy Check and finishing with an Energy Check each time. And, of course, do more if you're moved to! Ideally, I'd like you to do all seven series in order every day. You can do them all at once, or throughout the day, on their own or as a warm-up to the Sugar Savvy Power Workout. I've given you some directions about how many times you should do each movement (in most cases, I suggest doing the shout-out twice and the movement as many times as matches the shout-out). But don't feel restricted to these numbers—**move and shout for as long as it feels good!** In particular, you can do the Energy Check any time and as many times as you'd like— whether as part of your workout or just on its own, any time you need a little pick-me-up. Works better than a candy bar any day! Each series takes only 1 to 2 minutes—but *the natural high you'll get from this simple routine will last all day.* This is the energy that my name—High Voltage—represents!

Make Your Moving Affirmations Really Count!

Here are a few "rules" that will help make your Moving Affirmations even more powerful:

* Perform each movement and shout-out (except the warm-up and Energy Checks) in a rotation: facing forward, to the side, to the back, to the side, and then to the front again. When you face forward and back, really shout your affirmation out loud while you're doing the movement. When you're facing each side, really emphasize and exaggerate your movement while you silently think the affirmations powerfully in your mind.

* Bring all your star power to bear when you perform your Moving Affirmations; it's important to really BELIEVE in yourself and your ability to kick sugar and self-doubt out of your life for good.

* Do your affirmations in front of a mirror, so you can see your form and really talk directly *to* yourself. Some women find this a little uncomfortable as they try to avoid looking in mirrors. But part of loving, forgiving, and empowering yourself is *liking* yourself and that most certainly includes being able to like what you see in the mirror! If you have to, start small, by using a mirror that isn't full length. But eventually I want you to be able to perform these Moving Affirmations in front of a full-length mirror and LOVE what you see!

Warm-up: Positive Energy In

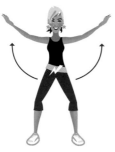 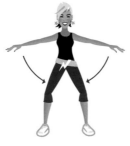 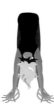

Step 1. Stand tall with your arms at your sides. Inhale and lift your arms out to the side, making a big circle and saying "Positive energy in."

Step 2. Exhale and bring your arms down to your side, saying, "Negative energy out." Repeat steps 1 and 2 five times.

Step 3. The last time you exhale your negative energy out, bend forward at the waist and reach down toward the floor.

Warm-up: Marching

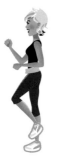

Movement: March in place for about 20 steps in each direction as you rotate (facing front, side, back, side).

Shout-out (twice): *"I am happy! I am healthy! All I need is within me now!"*

Start: Do an Energy Check!

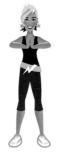 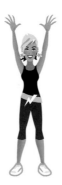 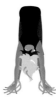

Step 1. Stand tall, feet hip-width apart. Clap at your chest.

Step 2. Reach both arms up as high as you can, shouting *whooo!* Then clap at your chest again.

Step 3. Reach down toward the floor. Then clap at your chest again. Repeat steps 2 and 3 ten times.

Affirmation Series 1: I Am the Master of My Fate! It's Never Too Late!

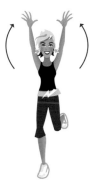

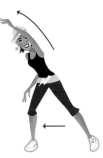

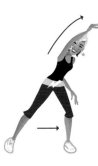

Movement: Step 1. Step to the right with your right foot and tap with your left foot while reaching up to the right with your left arm.

Step 2: Step to the left with your left foot and tap with your right foot while reaching up to the left with your right arm. Repeat steps 1 and 2 four times.

Shout-out (twice): *"I am the master of my fate! It's never too late!"*

Movement: Step 1. Jump and kick back your right foot, while raising your arms up.

Step 2 (not pictured). Jump and kick back your left foot, while raising your arms up. Repeat steps 1 and 2 four times.

Shout-out (twice): *"I am happy! I am healthy! My energy is up!"*

Repeat both sets of movements and shout-outs as you rotate to the side, back, and side.

Affirmation Series 2: I Am Strong And Powerful!

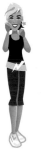

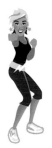

Step 3. Switch sides: Jump to the left. Step forward with your left foot while twisting your body to the right and punching forward with your left fist. Repeat four times.

Shout-out (twice): *"I am happy! I am healthy! I am strong and powerful!"*

Movement: Do an Energy Check! (see page 220)

Repeat both sets of movements and shout-outs as you rotate to the side, back, and side.

Movement: Step 1. Start in boxing stance. Stand with knees slightly bent, right foot in front, and arms in front of you making fists.

Step 2. Step forward with your right foot while twisting your body to the left and punching forward with your right fist. Repeat four times.

Affirmation Series 3: Rock! Roll! Free Your Soul!

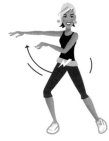 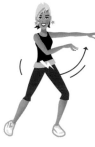 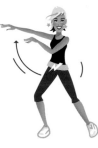

Movement: Step 1. Start facing forward with your feet a little more than hip-width apart, toes pointing out. Bend your right knee, rock your hips to the right, and swing your arms to the right, up to waist height.

Step 2. Bend your left knee, rock your hips to the left, and swing your arms to the left, up to waist height. Repeat steps 1 and 2 eight times.

Step 3. Rock your hips faster and swing your arms up higher and higher, about eight times. Then repeat steps 1 to 3 as you rotate to the side, back, and side.

Shout-out (four times):
"Rock! Roll! Free your soul!"

Affirmation Series 4: Nothing Can Stop Me!

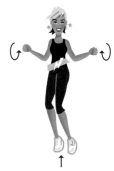 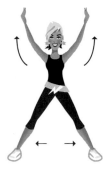

Movement: Pretend that you're jumping rope for about 20 jumps in each direction as you rotate (facing front, side, back, side).

Shout-out (twice): *"I am happy! I am healthy and nothing can stop me!"*

Movement: Do 20 jumping jacks, while counting from 1 to 20 loudly and proudly, in each direction as you rotate (facing front, side, back, side).

Affirmation Series 5: I Am the Best! And I Deserve the Best!

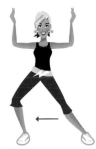

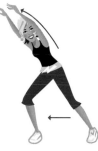

Movement: Step 1. Step to the right, with your arms open like goalposts, elbows bent and fingers pointing to the sky.

Step 2 (above, right). Bring your feet together, closing your arms but keeping your elbows bent and fingers pointing up.

Step 3 (not pictured). Step to the left, with your arms open like goalposts. Then bring your feet together, closing your arms. Repeat steps 1 through 3 six times.

Shout-out (twice): *"I am happy! I am healthy! I am the best! And I deserve the best!"*

Movement: Step 1. Step to the right with your right foot and tap with your left foot while reaching up and to the right with both arms.

Step 2 (not pictured). Step to the left with your left foot and tap with your right foot while reaching up and to the left with both arms. Repeat steps 1 and 2 four times.

Shout-out (twice): *"Reach, reach, reach for the stars!"*

Repeat both sets of movements and shout-outs as you rotate to the side, back, and side.

Affirmation Series 6: I Am Number One!

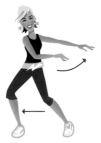

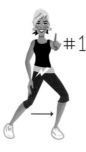

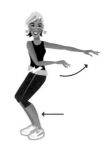

Movement: Step 1: Step to the right, twisting your body and raising your arms to the left.

Step 2 (not pictured). Step to the left, twisting your body and raising your arms to the right. Repeat steps 1 and 2 twice, while you say "I am happy! I am healthy!"

Step 3. Continue to twist your body to the left and right. Point to yourself while you say "I am" and make a #1 sign with your left hand while you say "number one!" Repeat steps 1 through 3.

Movement: Step 1. Jump to the right, feet together, twisting your body and swinging your arms to the left.

Step 2 (not pictured). Jump to the left, feet together, twisting your body and swinging your arms to the right. Repeat steps 1 and 2 eight times.

Shout-out (twice): *"Jump! Shout! Let it out!"*

Repeat both sets of movements and shout-outs as you rotate to the side, back, and side.

Affirmation Series 7: Pump It Up!

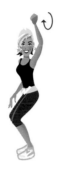
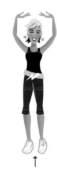

Movement: **Step 1.** Jump and pump your fist in a circle (think *Jersey Shore*!) with your right arm eight times.

Step 2 (not pictured). Jump and pump your fist in a circle with your left arm eight times. Repeat steps 1 and 2 as you rotate to the side, back, and side.

Shout out: *"Pump! Pump! Pump it up!"*

Movement: Jump up with your arms up, "raising the roof," about four times in each direction as you rotate (facing front, side, back, side).

Shout-out: *"Jump! Jump! Jump it higher!"*

Finish: Do an Energy Check!

Do an Energy Check! (see page 220)

THE POWER WORKOUT

Sugar Savvy Sisters are strong—inside and out! Most of this book has focused on building your mental muscles and strengthening your resolve to say NO THANK YOU to the sugar pushers and take control of your life by changing what you want. Now, we're going to work on the OUTSIDE and make those beautiful muscles shapely and strong so you can literally take on the world!

Strength training is an essential part of the Sugar Savvy solution. For one, lean, toned muscles make you look Fit, Fab, and Fierce! More importantly, especially for those who have sugar addictions, when you exercise, your brain pumps out lots of feel-good endorphins (the same ones food used to give you) to give you a **far healthier High Voltage high!** Exercise is also a natural mood booster, so you can fight the blues, the blahs, jealousy, and other emotional issues without wanting to reach for food! Finally, strength training gives you loads of energy! Think about it. The stronger you are, the easier everything is. You can bound up and down the stairs, carry groceries, shake your hips at Zumba class, and STILL have tons of energy left over!

Lean muscle tissue also helps keep your blood sugar in check. Every time you move your muscles, they need energy. When you make them work hard—like strength training does—they use a lot of glucose (i.e., blood sugar) to get the work done. Research also shows that the more muscle you have, the less likely you are to become diabetic. In one study from the University of California, Los Angeles, researchers examined health records from more than 13,600 men and women over 6 years and found that for every 10 percent increase in the ratio of lean muscle mass to total body weight, the risk of insulin resistance dropped 11 percent and the risk of developing prediabetes or diabetes dropped 12 percent. THAT'S HUGE!

Time to Make Some Muscle!

I designed this workout to hit and condition every muscle from head to toe. The goal is to firm all those muscles that may have gone flabby from disuse and to send your energy levels soaring. If you never strength-trained because you didn't want to get "bulky," don't worry, you won't! This program isn't designed to make you a bodybuilder; it's designed to build a better body through lots of repetitions, not by pumping heavy weights.

This workout is based on classic fitness movements that you may already be familiar with. It's completely straightforward, without any gimmicks or complex, hard-to-remember moves. The magic of this workout comes from the combination of these exercises and how they are ordered to systematically hit every muscle in your body.

You can do this simple routine *as often as you feel moved to.* Once you begin this routine (during Week 3 of the Sugar Savvy plan), I suggest that you start with one set once a week and **build up to doing the entire routine every day.** Yes, I said *every day.* Remember, this isn't about building bulging biceps. This is about strengthening your body and making your muscles firm and toned as well as beating stress and boosting your mood, so it's easier to change what you want. Your body is made to squat and lunge and reach and pull and push *every day!* You don't need a day of rest from this kind of activity. You need to do it as often as you can so you can keep moving and have tons of energy for the rest of your life! If you get bored doing this same routine every day, feel free to mix it up with other workouts. No matter what you do, however, **move your body every single day**, even when you're not strength training.

The Sugar Savvy Solution Moves

Many of these moves use an elastic resistance band to provide resistance. You can buy these bands at Target, Walmart, Amazon.com, or nearly any large department store. Start with the lowest resistance that feels comfortable to you. As you get stronger, you can add resistance by shortening the band. You may also use dumbbells where indicated with an asterisk. A pair of 5- and 10-pound dumbbells will do the trick.

You'll also need a sturdy chair, preferably without arms. You can also use a fitness ball (also called a Swiss ball), if you want an additional challenge (because fitness balls are inherently wobbly, your muscles will be forced to work just to keep you balanced while you perform your moves). Look for one that allows you to have a 90-degree bend in your legs when you sit on it. Most manufacturers also offer size guides that indicate which size ball is best for your height.

Do the prescribed number of repetitions for each move, then immediately move to the next exercise. Remember to exhale as you are working your muscles and to inhale when you return to the starting position.

Warm-up: Begin by standing tall, knees slightly bent. Perform neck rolls and shoulder rolls for 30 to 60 seconds.

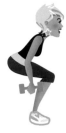

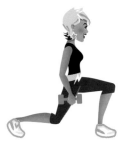

Squats:* Stand with your feet slightly apart, arms at your sides. (If you are using dumbbells, simply hold one in each hand.) Keeping your back straight, bend your knees as if you were going to sit in a chair, and drop your hips until your thighs are near parallel to the floor (pictured). (You can raise your arms straight out in front of you for balance.) Return to the starting position and squeeze your glutes. Repeat 10 times.

Note: Be especially careful to keep good form doing squats if you have any knee issues. Skip them if they really hurt.

Lunges:* Stand tall, feet slightly apart, knees slightly bent, with your arms at your sides. (If you are using dumbbells, simply hold one in each hand.) Take a giant step forward with your left leg and bend your knees so that your left thigh is parallel to the floor and your right knee drops toward the floor, right heel raised (pictured). Push back to the starting position, squeezing your glutes. Repeat 10 times. Switch sides.

Note: Lunges are an advanced move that you may not be able to do right out of the gate, particularly if you are new to strength training or are carrying some extra pounds that make it challenging. If that is you, wait a month or two to try them. Be especially careful if you have knee issues. Remember, it doesn't matter where you start—it's where you're going!

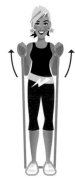

Biceps curls:* Stand on the center of the resistance band, feet slightly apart, arms at your sides, grasping the band with your palms facing forward so the band is taut. Keep your abs tight and your back straight. Bend your elbows and pull the band until your hands are up by your shoulders (pictured). Return to the starting position. Repeat 15 times.

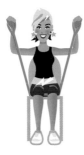

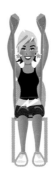

Shoulder presses:* **Step 1.** Sit in a chair with the band looped under the chair seat. Grasp the ends of the band in your hands and raise your arms out to the sides, elbows bent (in a goalpost position), palms facing forward.

Step 2. Extend your arms, bringing your hands together overhead. Return to the starting position. Repeat 15 times.

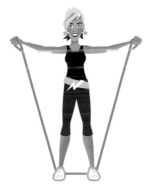

Lateral raises:* Stand on the center of the band, feet slightly apart, arms at your sides, grasping the band with your palms facing one another. Keeping a slight bend in your elbows, raise both arms out to the sides until they are parallel to the floor (pictured). Return to the starting position. Repeat 15 times.

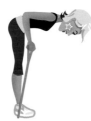

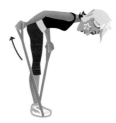

Triceps kickbacks:* **Step 1.** Stand on the center of the band, feet slightly apart, holding the ends at your waist, elbows bent. Keeping your back straight, bend forward from the hips. Pull the ends of the band up to about waist level, elbows at your ribcage.

Step 2. Extend your right arm straight back, keeping your elbows close to your side, pressing your palm toward the ceiling. Return to start. Repeat with your left arm. Alternating sides, repeat 15 times per side.

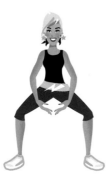

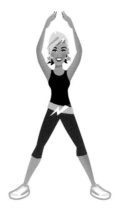

Pliés: Step 1. Stand tall, feet wider than shoulder-width apart, with your toes turned out and your heels in line with your shoulders. Bend your knees and bring your hands in front of you with your elbows slightly bent, fingers pointing to the floor.

Step 2. Raise your hands overhead while straightening your legs. Return to start. Repeat 10 times.

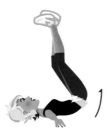

Lower ab lifts: Lie flat on the floor with your arms extended out to the side, palms down. Keeping your knees slightly bent and your ankles crossed, lift your legs toward the ceiling (pictured). Contract your abs and lift your butt off the floor. Return to start. Repeat 20 times.

Shake It Up

I honestly never grow tired of this workout because it's just part of my life and who I am! I do squats while I'm brushing my teeth and biceps curls while I'm watching a bit of TV in the evening. But I understand that for women not accustomed to weaving workouts into their daily lives, a strength-training routine can start to feel, well, routine. That's when it's time to shake things up!

Three weeks into the Sugar Savvy program, I busted out a box of glow wands during a meeting with our Sugar Savvy Sisters and we did our workout to music with whirling, flashing wands in a dimmed room. Was it silly? You bet! Was it fun? You bet! That's the point. This is supposed to be energizing! This is supposed to be a celebration of your fabulous self! So get creative! Pump up your favorite tunes, turn down the lights, grab some glow sticks, and get going! Even better, invite some friends over and make it a power workout party! When you make working out fun, it's never work!

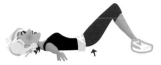

Pelvic tilt: Lie flat on the floor with your arms extended out to the side, palms down, and your knees bent, feet flat on the floor. Contract your abs and push your pelvis forward about 2 inches off the floor, keeping the small of your back on the floor (pictured). Return to start. Repeat 20 times.

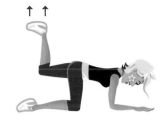

Butt lifts: Get on all fours with your arms bent so your forearms are resting on the floor. Keeping your left knee bent, raise your left leg so that your left thigh and the sole of your left foot are parallel to the ceiling. Press your left foot up as though you want to put a footprint on the ceiling (pictured). Return to start. Repeat 10 times. Switch sides.

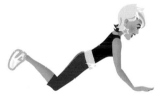

Push-ups: Assume a modified push-up position, with your knees bent, ankles crossed, arms extended with your hands on the floor slightly wider apart than your shoulders (pictured). Bend your elbows and lower your chest toward the floor until your arms are bent 90 degrees. Return to start. Do as many as you can. Work up to three sets of 20. (Or, if this is too easy, you can instead do traditional push-ups with your legs extended.)

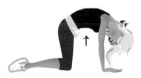

Angry cat: Get on all fours, arms straight, hands on the floor slightly wider apart than your shoulders. Pull your navel toward your spine while arching your back and dropping your head slightly forward (pictured). Return to start. Repeat 10 times.

Keep It Going! Sugar Savvy Living Forever

Congratulations! You did it! You educated yourself. You dedicated yourself. You got your **weight down** and your **energy up**! Give yourself a pat on the back. Then get your boots back on and dig in for round two.

I can hear you now: ***What?! Round two?? What do you mean, round two??*** That's right. I said round two. Look: I've been around for a long time. I've seen every diet under the sun come and go . . . and then come and go again! The Sugar Savvy solution is a complete lifestyle change, but if you stop now, you run the risk of treating it like every other diet out there. **That will not work.**

We've all seen it. A book comes out. The media rally around it. People lose weight and sing its praises. Problem solved, right? WRONG. This problem has been around since we began processing our food; it's not ending anytime soon. Really. Over the decades, I've watched the diet and fitness industry become bigger as *we're* getting bigger! So clearly something is not working. It's the "I did it. I'm cured. Life goes on as normal" mentality! People stop and get sloppy and forgetful.

The same can happen here. You can forget that you don't like sugary, salty CRAP foods anymore. You can start thinking, "Oh, it's such and such's birthday tomorrow. I HAVE to have some cake. It's so-and-so's baby shower Sunday; I'll need to eat chips and cookies." Before you know it, you're back to bingeing and being a food addict. It's like the alcoholic who says after 8 weeks sober, "I'm cured! I can have a little wine with dinner." And she can. Until she wakes up in a strange bed after a blackout. Sure, that's an extreme example. But it's 100 percent true. One of our Sugar Savvy Sisters confided in me that she's struggling terribly with being a "foodie" as well as a Sugar Savvy Sister for this very reason. She does well for a while and thinks she can manage it and then, before you know it, she spirals out of control again. Once an addict, always an addict, people! The only cure is not taking that first bite or sip.

This isn't just a book. This isn't just a diet. This is a real, live way to live—with *you* in control, NOT your trigger foods and sugar. Just because you're turning the final pages doesn't mean it's over! FAR from it! You're just getting started!

ROUND TWO: CYCLE FOR SUCCESS

So what should you do now? Soupalicious! If you find yourself slipping and "forgetting" you don't like CRAP foods too often or just feel like Sugar Savvy living is not yet second nature, you need another "reboot." It's time to really **double down** to make this big lifestyle change stick! Now is the time to consider doing the Palate Cleanse again, kick those trigger foods to the curb, and drink that water! This is especially important if you have yet to achieve your goal because it will put you in the FAST LANE on the highway to Fit, Fab, and Fierce Drive. Double down and hit the gas pedal!

It's not just Soupalicious Soup and the eating components you'll be doing again, but fully focusing on your affirmations and your attitude of gratitude and forgiveness, as well as expanding your workout possibilities. Certainly, you don't have to revisit every detail of the plan. If you've created your recharging station and have already performed all your sugar shockers, there's no need to redo them. There are certainly aspects that you have down pat at this point. But let's face it, you digested a LOT of information these past 6 weeks and have made an ENORMOUS sea change in your life! There will be a few things that slip off the radar or that you never fully got the hang of! Now that you're familiar with this program, you'll be able to dive in with even more focus and attention the second time around and really concentrate on those aspects of the Sugar Savvy solution that didn't stick as well as you would have liked the first time around.

> It's time to **double down** to make this big lifestyle change stick!

Take the time to fine-tune your affirmations. Write some new ones that reflect where you are now and where you are going. Look at your workout. You should always be doing your **loud and proud** Moving Affirmations, but what about the rest of it? Have you advanced your strength training so you're now doing three sets of each move? Have you incorporated dumbbells? Have you tried any NEW ways to move your body? ***Dig in and go for it!***

Honestly, even after all these years, I'm still learning new things and refining my own Sugar Savvy living. Up until recently, I had never really cooked! I ate well, but I bought a lot of food instead of making it myself. As I refined the meal plan, I started making my own food and I can't believe how wonderful and easy it is!

As you cycle back through the program, take the time to go those extra miles to **be fully prepared at all times!** That's another one that I'm still learning! Just the other day, I took a group of my

Energy Up! girls out to the Museum of Natural History and I broke RULE #1! *I was not prepared!* They were having a global food exhibit, so I thought there would be amazing food there. WRONG! The healthiest thing I could find was a falafel in a pita. I ate the falafel, lettuce, and tomatoes and dumped the pita. It was difficult. Nothing was really Sugar Savvy approved. So I made the best choice I could. **Don't get stuck without your food!**

Our dietitian Jessica has the best advice for being prepared, which I can boil down to one word: PLAN! Sit down at the beginning of the week and plan out your Power Meals and Power Drinks so that you have everything you need in order to put them together quickly and easily. If you're eating grains, make one large batch in the beginning of the week, so you can just nuke them as needed. Do the same for beans, starchy vegetables, or even roasted or steamed veggies that you like. If it's easier for you, you can also "double up" on one aspect. For example, if making the Power Drinks is pretty easy for you, you can always have two of them in a day and have just three Power Meals. Keep working to find a system that is easy and automatic for you!

If you have not yet stocked up on great "take-along" accessories like insulated lunch bags, thermoses, and food containers, *definitely do this now!* Sugar Savvy living is WAY easier to accomplish if you bring your Power Meals along with you during the day rather than put them together with what you find out "in the world."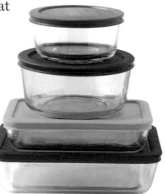

Get creative! So many eating situations can catch you off guard! There's going to the movies (it seems to be written somewhere that you cannot see a movie without chewing on some sort of food!). There are ball games. It's always somebody's birthday. **Take your food with you.** You can take a snack bag of baby carrots to the movies or ball game. You can take a Power Drink in a to-go cup. When you have Sugar Savvy food with you, you will never be tempted by foods you no longer want, because you have what you want!

> Keep working to find a system that is **easy and automatic** for you.

Keep those boots to the ground and keep marching to the Sugar Savvy drumbeat! And when these 6 weeks are through, DO IT AGAIN until you hit your goal! That's right. Keep cycling through the Sugar Savvy plan, each time digging a little deeper, learning a little more, trying new things, making new affirmations, until you hit your goal and STAY THERE (and even then, you need to stay the course for life, though you don't need to keep cycling through the plan). Be happy and energized by all your success, but don't look at it as "Now I am cured!"

That being said, remember that you don't need to feel stuck with the Power Meal formulas or the foods we listed in Chapter 10 for the rest of your life. If the formulas are working for you and you've discovered some new favorite veggies and whole grains you could eat every day, great! They can continue to be your guide to creating nutritious, balanced Sugar Savvy meals that energize you. But if the Sugar Savvy solution has inspired you to be even more adventurous and you're itching to try some new foods (I've recently discovered "pastas" made from beans, for instance, which are filling and fantastic!), GO FOR IT! As long as you stay away from sugary processed foods, you will still keep losing weight and feeling great! By now, you should have a pretty good idea of what foods are Sugar Savvy and how (and how much!) to eat them. Refer back to the 10 Sugar Savvy power points on page 142 for more general guidelines on how you can keep eating Sugar Savvy.

And also remember that you should always feel Fit, Fabulous, and Fierce while you're eating the Sugar Savvy way. If you don't, and you really aren't sneaking any CRAP, then you may need to eat more food. Everyone's calorie needs are different, and it's possible you just need a little more fuel to keep your **energy up**! The Sugar Savvy Meal Plan presented in this book is designed for the calorie needs of average-height, mostly sedentary adult women. If you've lost weight or really ramped up your activity level, go ahead and add a little more to your plate—just remember to stick to Sugar Savvy foods and don't use this as an excuse to load up and go to town (even on the healthy stuff!). Most people OVEREAT—a lot!

Keep marching! The more you dig in, the more you will protect what you have fought so hard to change because it will become so precious and important. You'll feel so great and look so fabulous, you will **defend** it with all you've got! I protect my sleep and hydration and I'm absolutely vigilant about what I put in my mouth because I know where I'll end up if I don't! The more you invest, the more you'll get out of the plan, and the more permanent all these positive changes will become! ***The Sugar Savvy solution works.*** Just like Alcoholics Anonymous, the program works if you work the program, one day at a time.

LESSONS FROM THE SUGAR SAVVY SISTERHOOD

If our Sugar Savvy Sisters could give you just one word of advice to be successful, it would be this: **Prepare!** We're so used to eating on the run, grabbing and going, drive-thru ordering, and mindlessly picking up whatever food happens to be "convenient," that it takes a bit of planning and preparation to make the transition to Sugar Savvy eating. Nearly all of our Sugar Savvy Sisters took the following steps to be successful:

> The more you invest, **the more you'll get** out of the plan.

- **Plan ahead:** Plan your meals and snacks and pack them up the night before a long work or school day. "I live in a big city, so if I don't plan ahead I'm vulnerable to a lot of bad choices. I have my blender ready in the morning to make healthy shakes. I plan my veggies and protein for lunch. I know what I'll have for a snack. It takes a lot of the stress out of the day because my good choices are already made," says Nancy Barthold, 51.

- **Equip yourself:** Invest in some tools like insulated lunch bags, ice packs, and thermoses that will allow you to toss your meals and snacks into an easy-to-carry container and take them with you wherever you go! They have designer ones now—they could even match your shoes! "I used to carry packaged crackers in my bag. Now, with a cute little cooler bag, I can carry cauliflower and have a healthier, satisfying crunch!" says Sugar Savvy Sister (literally—she's my sister!) Bonnie O'Gallagher, 62.

- **Make large batches:** Chop up your veggies in one fell swoop and store them in your fridge. Make large batches of grains and beans early in the week. Make a double batch of the Power Drink recipe and store half for later. The easier you make it on yourself to have what you need on hand, the more likely you are to eat as planned. "Monday is my cooking day. I buy and chop everything. I cook everything. I measure it out into meal-sized containers. I label it. And I'm good to go for the week!" says Sugar Savvy Sister Lisa Brooks, 49.

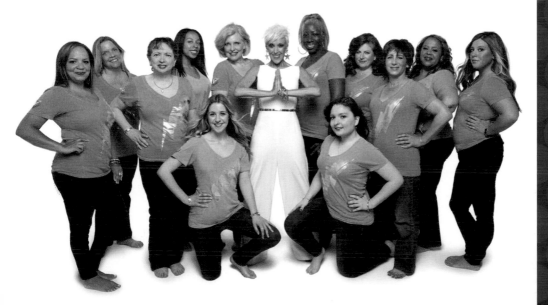

OUR SUGAR SAVVY LEGACY

Revolutions may start with a single person's ideas, but the war is won by an army. There is strength in numbers, and right now you're FAR outnumbered by the industrial food complex! But the tide is turning. The drumbeat is growing ever louder. People across the nation are starting to rise up and say ENOUGH! We are truly FED UP! That, by the way, is the name of a recent documentary co-produced by my longtime client and dear friend Katie Couric, which really rings the alarm bell on this ENORMOUS problem. It's well worth watching (and I'd say that even if Energy Up! weren't featured in it!).

> We are **vital, alive, energetic** Sugar Savvy Sisters!

The Sugar Savvy solution is the answer to this problem. It's creating a sisterhood that LITERALLY takes the message to the 'hood! Take this message to your family. Take this message to your friends. Take this message to your neighborhood and find compatriots who will join you in the Sugar Savvy revolution!

We need to shop and speak with our wallets. We need to cook. We need to take our **tremendous energy** and focus it to educate the country to the fact that SUGAR is America's #1 DRUG! As our self-confidence grows larger, our bodies get smaller. Our eyes light up with ENERGY and KNOWLEDGE and we shine that light on the world around us! One of the coolest things about teaching the Energy Up! girls how to live Sugar Savvy was to see the ripple effect they had on their peers, their teachers, and their parents.

Fifty years from now, I want people to say, "There was a woman named High Voltage at the beginning of this." I devoted my life to this cause. I want Sugar Savvy living to be my legacy. I want it to be

OUR legacy. That means we have to stay fully dedicated to it no matter what life throws our way. And life will throw lots of s*** our way!

Throughout your life, you will go through things you cannot control. That's inevitable! ***But what you eat and think you CAN control!*** No matter what else happens, you can get happier and healthier every single day! Turn on and tune in to the UNIVERSAL ENERGY all around us.

Right now, every second we live the Sugar Savvy way, we are doing what many think is impossible, ***but it is clearly possible***! We are not average. We do not want to be normal—which in this country means being sick, overweight, and depressed. We want to be EXTRAORDINARY! We are vital, alive, energetic Sugar Savvy Sisters!

Do not let life pull you off course. Even after you reach and maintain your goal weight, the Soupalicious Palate Cleanse and Sugar Savvy Meal Plan are there for you. The star points and power points are there to help you shine. They should be your guiding light, always!

- You can get hydrated.
- You can move your body every single day!
- You can be grateful for all you have.
- You can stay under 24 grams of added sugar each day!
- You can announce your affirmations loudly and proudly.
- You can eat Sugar Savvy approved.
- You can do this.
- You ARE doing this—today and every day!

HAVE A FIT, FAB, AND FIERCE SUGAR SAVVY DAY!!!!!

APPENDIX A: THE SUGAR SAVVY STARTER KIT

If you choose to follow the sample workweek's plan in Chapter 5, here's what you'll need to get. It may seem like a long list, but don't be overwhelmed! In this first week, you'll be stocking up on staples and seasonings that will last for some time. Consider this your Sugar Savvy Starter Kit. Don't forget to make adjustments to your list if you make substitutions in some of your meals or if you're cooking for more than one person. Note that this list is organized according to where you'll most likely find items in your grocery store.

Beans/Peas/Legumes*

- Black beans, dried (1 small bag)
- Chickpeas or garbanzo beans, dried (1 small bag)
- Kidney beans, dried (1 small bag)

Note: You can also choose to use canned beans, if you prefer; choose those with the lowest sodium content and BPA-free cans when possible.

Canned Goods

- Quartered artichoke hearts (choose those with the lowest sodium content) (1 small can or jar)
- Tuna, canned in water (5-oz can)
- Water chestnuts (1 small can)
- Sun-dried tomatoes (1 package)

Note: Look for low-sodium versions and choose BPA-free cans when possible.

Grains/"Carbs"

- Brown rice (1 small bag)

- Sprouted whole grain or 100% whole grain bread (no sugar added) (1 loaf)

- Sprouted whole grain or 100% whole grain pasta, such as buckwheat (soba), quinoa, or brown rice pasta (1 small package)

- Sprouted whole grain or 100% whole grain English muffins (no sugar added) (1 small package)

- Steel-cut oatmeal (1 can or package)

- 100% whole grain, high-fiber, nut- or seed-based crackers (no sugar added and low in sodium), such as Mary's Gone Crackers (1 package)

- Barley (hulled or "hull-less"—not pearled) (1 small bag)

Note: If any of these are trigger foods for you, skip them and substitute a different grain or some starchy vegetables instead.

Time-Saving Tips

To save time during the hectic workweek, try these tips:

* Roast the veggies you'll use during the week (sweet potatoes, Brussels sprouts, broccoli) ahead of time. Wash, peel, trim, and chop them into 1-inch pieces. Mist with olive oil and bake them in a 350°F oven for 20 to 35 minutes. Check on them periodically. You may want to toss the veggies to help them cook evenly. If they appear dry, you can mist with a little more oil. The sweet potatoes will take longer to cook than the other veggies. You can also try coconut oil as an alternative to the olive oil. You will want to melt it first and then toss the veggies in it.

* If using dried beans (our preferred method), soak them overnight and cook them the next day. If using canned beans, rinse them thoroughly, soak them for 30 minutes, and then rinse again before using to avoid excess sodium.

* Make some wheat berries and brown rice ahead of time as well. Be aware that some forms of whole grains require soaking overnight before cooking, so read the cooking instructions carefully.

* In general, anything that you make ahead of time (oats, roasted veggies, dried beans, wheat berries, brown rice, grilled chicken, etc.) will keep in the fridge for 1 to 5 days, so plan accordingly. Check foodsafety.gov for more information on proper food storage.

Produce

- Arugula (one 5-oz package)
- Asparagus (6 spears)
- Avocado (3)
- Baby spinach (two 5-oz packages)
- Bell pepper, green (1) (Note that different colored bell peppers are all interchangeable.)
- Bell pepper, red (3 or 4) (Note that different colored bell peppers are all interchangeable.)
- Bell pepper, yellow (1 or 2) (Note that different colored bell peppers are all interchangeable.)
- Broccoli (3½ cups)
- Brussels sprouts (1 small bag) (Note that this can be used in Grilled Veggie Salad if desired, in place of the mushrooms or asparagus.)
- Carrots (1 small bunch)
- Corn (1 fresh ear or 1 small bag frozen)
- Cucumber (1 small)
- Eggplant (1 small)
- Garlic (1 head)
- Grape tomatoes (2 pints)
- Green onions/scallions (1 small bunch)
- Kale (1 bunch, about 3 cups)
- Mushrooms, sliced (1 small package)
- Red onion (1 small)
- Shallots (1 small)
- Spring mix (one 5 oz package)
- Tomato (1 small)

- Zucchini (2 or 3 small)
- Banana (3, about 6 in. long)
- Blueberries (1 pint)
- Grapes, seedless red (1 small bunch)
- Oranges (4, about 2½–3 in. in diameter)
- Pineapple chunks (3 cups)
- Tofu, light, extra firm, fortified with calcium and vitamins D and B12, preferably organic and non-GMO such as Nosaya Organic Firm Tofu Plus (one 14-oz package)

Optional: The following items are included in this week's sample menu, but in small amounts. You can easily sub in other fruits and vegetables should you choose not to purchase these.

- Snow peas (½ cup)
- Swiss chard (1 small bunch)
- Mango (1 small)
- Peach (1 small)
- Basil (1 small bunch)
- Parsley (1 small bunch)

When to Go Organic

I always go with organic milk products, meats, and of course fruits and veggies to make sure I avoid any pesticides or other potential toxins. It's not required by any means. The one time I really recommend that you try to prioritize organic produce is when buying fruits and veggies that are notoriously pesticide ridden. Here is the Environmental Working Group's list of the "Dirty Dozen." Eat organic varieties of these foods when possible. If you're shopping at local farmers' markets, the farmers may not be 100 percent organic, but their produce is still often a wonderful choice because it's locally grown and fewer nutrients are lost in transit.

1. apples
2. celery
3. sweet bell peppers
4. peaches
5. strawberries
6. nectarines (imported)
7. grapes
8. spinach
9. lettuce
10. cucumbers
11. blueberries (domestic)
12. potatoes

Condiments, Oils, Nuts, and Seeds

- Salsa (no sugar added)
- Tahini
- Dijon mustard
- Red wine vinegar
- Extra virgin olive oil
- Coconut oil
- Almonds (unsalted)
- Walnuts (unsalted)
- Flaxseed meal
- Chia seeds

Dairy and Eggs

- Eggs
- Fat-free plain Greek yogurt
- Low-fat (or fat-free) feta cheese
- Low-fat (or fat-free) goat cheese (or other cheese slices)
- Low-fat no-sodium-added cottage cheese
- Skim milk (if desired, to make oatmeal with)
- Unsweetened nonfat soy milk made from whole soy beans such as Organic Valley Unsweetened Soy Milk or almond milk with added protein such as So Delicious Unsweetened Almond Plus 5X (fortified with calcium and vitamins D and B12)

Note: Choose organic if possible.

APPENDIX B: THE SUGAR SAVVY PANTRY

Because the Sugar Savvy Meal Plan is designed so you can customize it for what works for you, there are no set menus or shopping lists. That being said, the more you can stock your pantry, freezer, and fridge with REAL FOOD, the easier it will be for you to create delicious Power Meals and Power Drinks. Here's a list of some things you may want to have on hand to get started.

Most of the items on the list have a fairly long shelf life. In the case of perishable items (marked with an asterisk), don't buy too much or they will go to waste. Breads and meats can be frozen, but the others are best when fresh. Also, buy small quantities of unfamiliar foods to start with—we want you to try new foods, but there's no need to choke it all down if you really don't like something on this list.

Fruits and Veggies*

Stock up on some of your favorite fruits and vegetables. Pick up some leafy greens like spinach, kale, collard greens, or Swiss chard. Grab additional non-starchy veggies in a variety of colors, such as carrots, bell peppers, and tomatoes. Add some sweet juicy fruits to snack on, including berries, apples, pears, grapes, and oranges. Experiment with less-familiar fruits and veggies, too; try eggplant, kohlrabi, pomegranate, kiwi, and much more. Check out the list of Vital Veggies in Chapter 10 for more ideas. (Choose organic if possible.)

Beans & Peas

- 1 or 2 bags dried beans of your choice (or no-sodium-added canned beans; choose BPA-free cans if possible, such as Eden Organic or Trader Joe's)
- Fresh or frozen green peas*
- Dried lentils

Carbs

Stock up on some whole grains, which can usually be found in the bulk food section of some grocery stores or in the aisle with rice and pasta. Be sure not to get "mixed" dishes that are microwaveable and contain other ingredients. You're going for the whole grain and nothing but the grain. Try these:

- Quinoa
- Wheat berries
- Brown or wild rice
- Sprouted whole grain or 100% whole grain bread* such as Alvarado St. Bakery, Rudi's Organic Bakery, or Ezekiel 4:9 (sprouted grain bread products are oftentimes frozen and can be stored longer at home that way, too!)
- Muesli (no sugar added), such as Familia No Added Sugar Swiss Muesli, Alpen All Natural Muesli, or Bob's Red Mill Old Country Style Muesli
- Steel-cut oats
- 100% whole grain, high-fiber nut- or seed-based crackers. such as Mary's Gone Crackers
- Sprouted whole grain or 100% whole grain pastas such as Ezekiel 4:9 Sprouted Wheat Spaghetti, Ancient Harvest Whole Grain Quinoa Pasta, Lundberg Family Farms Organic Brown Rice Pasta, or Eden Organic 100% Buckwheat Soba Noodles

Also, don't forget that starchy vegetables qualify as Supercharged Carbs in your Sugar Savvy Meal Plan. So stock up on sweet potatoes or squash, too—especially if whole grains are a trigger food for you.

Proteins

- 1 carton eggs* (choose organic if possible)

- Lean meats such as chicken, ground sirloin, or pork tenderloin* (choose organic if possible; for beef, choose grass-fed if possible) (to save on time, you can also purchase precooked meats; just look for ones that have been grilled or roasted, with no sauces that may contain added sugar)

- Fish/seafood (fresh or frozen)* (choose wild-caught if possible)

- Canned tuna (in water) (choose BPA-free cans if possible)

- Shelled edamame*, light tofu* such as Nasoya Organic Extra Firm Tofu Plus, or tempeh* such as Lightlife Organic Soy Tempeh (usually found in the refrigerated area near fresh produce) (tofu and tempeh should be made from whole soy beans and fortified with calcium and vitamin D and, ideally, B12) (choose organic and non-GMO if possible)

Fats

- Olive oil
- Coconut oil
- Flaxseed meal
- Avocados*

Milks & Yogurt

- Unsweetened shelf-stable soy milk or almond milk (fortified with calcium and vitamins D and B12) (look for almond milk with protein added such as So Delicious Unsweetened Almond Plus 5X and soy milk made from whole soy beans such as Organic Valley Unsweetened Soy Milk) (choose organic if possible)

- Fat-free plain Greek yogurt* such as Stonyfield, Wallaby, or Trader Joe's (choose organic if possible)

- Skim milk* (if you drink dairy) (choose organic if possible)

APPENDIX C: SUGAR SAVVY POWER MEAL FORMULAS

For easy reference, here's a "cheat sheet" listing all the Power Meal formulas. Post this on your fridge or bring it with you when you eat out! Please note that there are variations in serving sizes depending upon the individual food. Please refer to Chapter 10 for more details.

Vital Veggie Power Meal Formulas

Pure Protein

2 Veggies (2 cups raw or 1 cup cooked) **+ 1 Fat** (1 tsp oil; 1 Tbsp seeds; 6–10 nuts) **+ 2 Proteins** (2 oz; 2 eggs) **+ 1 Carb** (½ cup cooked; 1 slice) **+ 1 Fruit** (1 small or ½–1 cup)

You may substitute 2 Veggies for the 1 Fruit in this formula if desired.

Mean Bean

2 Veggies (2 cups raw or 1 cup cooked) **+ 1 Fat** (1 tsp oil; 1 Tbsp seeds; 6–10 nuts) **+ 2 Beans & Peas** (1 cup cooked)

Mix It Up

2 Veggies (2 cups raw or 1 cup cooked) **+ 1 Fat** (1 tsp oil; 1 Tbsp seeds; 6–10 nuts) **+ 1 Protein** (1 oz; 1 egg) **+ 1 Beans & Peas** (½ cup cooked) **+ 1 Carb** (½ cup cooked; 1 slice)

Supercharged Carb Power Meal Formulas

Pure Protein

1 Carb (½ cup cooked; 1 slice) **+ 1 Fat** (1 tsp oil; 1 Tbsp seeds; 6–10 nuts) **+ 2 Proteins** (2 oz; 2 eggs) **+ 1 Veggie** (1 cup raw or ½ cup cooked) **+ 1 Fruit** (1 small or ½–1 cup)

You may substitute 2 Veggies for the 1 Fruit in this formula if desired.
You may also substitute ½ Fruit for the 1 Veggie in this formula if desired.

Mean Bean

1 Carb (½ cup cooked; 1 slice) **+ 1 Fat** (1 tsp oil; 1 Tbsp seeds; 6–10 nuts)
+ 1 Protein (1 oz; 1 egg) **+ ½ Beans & Peas** (¼ cup cooked) **+ 2 Veggies**
(2 cups raw or 1 cup cooked)

You may substitute ½ Fruit for 1 of the 2 Veggies in this formula if desired.

Dairy Does It

1 Carb (½ cup cooked; 1 slice) **+ 1 Fat** (1 tsp oil; 1 Tbsp seeds; 6–10 nuts)
+ 1½ Milks & Yogurt (1½ cups milk; 9 oz yogurt) **+ ½ Fruit** (½ small or
¼ cup–½ cup)

You may substitute 1 Veggie for the ½ Fruit in this formula if desired.

Power Drink Formulas

Greek Goddess

½ cup fat-free plain Greek yogurt **+ 2 Veggies** (2 cups raw) **+ 1½ Fruits**
(1½ small or ¾–1½ cups) **+ 2 Fats** (2 tsp oil; 2 Tbsp seeds; 12–20 nuts)

Nondairy Delight

**1 cup unsweetened soy milk or 2 cups unsweetened almond milk
(fortified with calcium and vitamins D and B12) + 1 Veggie** (1 cup raw)
+ 2 Fruits (2 small or 1–2 cups) **+ 1 Protein** (1–3 oz light tofu fortified with
calcium and vitamins D and B12 or Voltage-approved protein powder, in
a portion that provides at least 7 g protein) **+ 1 Fat** (1 tsp oil; 1 Tbsp seeds;
6–10 nuts)

In the case of soy milk, choose one that has been made from fresh whole soy beans.
In the case of almond milk, choose one that has added protein.

Fruit and Veggie Refresher

1 cup water + 2 Veggies (2 cups raw) **+ 2 Fruits** (2 small or 1–2 cups) **+
2 Proteins** (2–6 oz tofu or Voltage-approved protein powder, in a portion
that provides at least 14 g protein) **+ 1 Fat** (1 tsp oil; 1 Tbsp seeds; 6–10 nuts)

You may increase or decrease the amount of water as desired.

NOTES

Part 1

Introduction

page ix, "... adults is now clinically obese." K. M. Flegal et al., "Prevalence of Obesity and Trends in the Distribution of Body Mass Index among US Adults, 1999–2010," JAMA 307, no. 5 (2012): 491–97. Available online: http://jama.ama-assn.org/content/307/5/491.

page ix, "... children are clinically obese." C. L. Ogden et al., "Prevalence of Obesity and Trends in Body Mass Index among US Children and Adolescents, 1999–2010," JAMA 307, no. 5 (2012): 483–90. Available online: http://jama.ama-assn.org/content/307/5/483.

page ix, "... with prediabetes." Centers for Disease Control and Prevention, "National Diabetes Fact Sheet: National Estimates and General Information on Diabetes and Prediabetes in the United States, 2011," Atlanta, GA: US Department of Health and Human Services, Centers for Disease Control and Prevention, 2011, http://www.cdc.gov/diabetes/pubs/factsheet11.htm#citation.

page xvi, "... 13 pounds per school year." "'Energy Up': A Novel Approach to the Weight Management of Inner-city Teens," *Journal of Adolescent Health* 40, no. 5 (May 2007): 474–76. Epub March 9, 2007.

Chapter 1

page 4, "... over the past 30 years?!" Caroline S. Fox et al., "Trends in the Incidence of Type 2 Diabetes Mellitus from the 1970s to the 1990s," *Circulation* 113 (2006): 2914–18. Published online before print June 19, 2006. doi: 10.1161/http://circ.ahajournals.org/content/113/25/2914.full.

page 5, "... limited cafeteria access." Paul M. Johnson and Paul J. Kenny, "Addiction-like Reward Dysfunction and Compulsive Eating in Obese Rats: Role of Dopamine D2 Receptors," *Nature Neuroscience 13, no. 5* (May 2010): 635–41. Published online March 28, 2010. doi: 10.1038/nn.2519, http://www.ncbi.nlm.nih.gov/pmc/articles/PMC2947358/.

page 6, "... 4,500 calories a day." D. E. Larsen et al., "Spontaneous Overfeeding with a 'Cafeteria Diet' in Men: Effects on 24-hour Energy Expenditure and Substrate Oxidation," *International Journal of Obesity and Related Metabolic Disorders 19, no. 5 (May 1995)*: 331–37. Available online: http://www.ncbi.nlm.nih.gov/pubmed/7647825.

page 6, "... brains of their unborn babies!" Jessica R. Gugusheff, Zhi Yi Ong, and Beverly S. Muhlhausler, "A Maternal 'Junk-food' Diet Reduces Sensitivity to the Opioid Antagonist Naloxone in Offspring Postweaning," Journal of the Federation of American Societies for Experimental Biology 27, no. 3 (March 2013): 1275–84. Published online before print December 11, 2012. doi: 10.1096/fj.12-217653, http://www.fasebj.org/content/27/3/1275.abstract.

page 12, "... story published in an academic journal." "'Energy Up': A Novel Approach to the Weight Management of Inner-city Teens," *Journal of Adolescent Health* 40, no. 5 (May 2007): 474–76. Epub March 9, 2007.

Chapter 2

page 22, "... the latest figures from the United States Department of Agriculture (USDA)." Hodan Farah Wells and Jean C. Buzby, "Dietary Assessment of Major Trends in U.S. Food Consumption, 1970-2005," Economic Information Bulletin No. EIB33,

March 2008. Available online: http://www.ers.usda.gov/publications/eib-economic-information-bulletin/eib33.aspx#.UqZBWCRgNhA

page 22, ". . . 88 grams or 22 teaspoons" Rachel K. Johnson et al., "Dietary Sugars Intake and Cardiovascular Health: A Scientific Statement from the American Heart Association," *Circulation* 120 (2009): 1011–20. Originally published online August 24, 2009. doi: 10.1161/CIRCULATIONAHA.109.192627. http://circ.ahajournals.org/content/120/11/1011.full.pdf.

page 22, ". . . enough to add 33⅓ pounds over the course of a year!" R. B. Ervin et al., "Consumption of Added Sugar among US Children and Adolescents, 2005–2008," NCHS data brief no. 87. Hyattsville, MD: National Center for Health Statistics, 2012. Available online: http://www.cdc.gov/nchs/data/databriefs/db87.pdf.

page 25, ". . . comes from processed foods," Kai Ryssdal, "Processed Foods Make 70 Percent of the US Diet," Marketplace, http://www.marketplace.org/topics/life/big-book/processed-foods-make-70-percent-us-diet.

page 25, ". . . through these meals and snacks!" R. B. Ervin and C. L. Ogden, "Consumption of Added Sugars among US Adults, 2005–2010," NCHS data brief no. 122. Hyattsville, MD: National Center for Health Statistics, 2013. Available online: http://www.cdc.gov/nchs/data/databriefs/db122.htm#ref6.

page 25, ". . . 25,000 right here in the United States." Dariush Mozaffarian et al., research presented at the American Heart Association's Epidemiology and Prevention/Nutrition, Physical Activity and Metabolism 2013 Scientific Sessions. Available online:http://newsroom.heart.org/news/180-000-deaths-worldwide-may-be-associated-with-sugary-soft-drinks.

page 28, ". . . at least 40 percent sugar!" "Some Breakfast Cereals Marketed to Kids Are More Than 50 Percent Sugar," *Consumer Reports*, November 2008.

page 35, ". . . (again, little wonder you can't eat just one!)." B. Wolfgang et al., "Relation of Addiction Genes to Hypothalamic Gene Changes Subserving Genesis and Gratification of a Classic Instinct, Sodium Appetite," *Proceedings of the National Academy of Sciences* (2011). doi:10.1073/pnas.1109199108.

page 35, ". . . heart attacks, stroke, and other heart disease." Saman Fahimi et al., research presented at the American Heart Association's Epidemiology and Prevention/Nutrition, Physical Activity and Metabolism 2013 Scientific Sessions. Available online: http://newsroom.heart.org/news/eating-too-much-salt-led-to-nearly-2-3-million-heart-related-deaths-worldwide-in-2010.

page 35, ". . . between 1/2 teaspoon and 3/4 teaspoon—a very small amount!" John Powles et al., research presented at the American Heart Association's Nutrition, Physical Activity and Metabolism and Cardiovascular Disease Epidemiology and Prevention 2013 Scientific Sessions. Available online: http://newsroom.heart.org/news/adults-worldwide-eat-almost-double-daily-aha-recommended-amount-of-sodium.

page 35, ". . . for your body to function properly—that's what I personally aim for." Centers for Disease Control and Prevention, "Americans Consume Too Much Sodium (Salt)," Atlanta, GA: U.S. Department of Health and Human Services, Centers for Disease Control and Prevention, 2011, http://www.cdc.gov/features/dssodium.

page 35, ". . . that's 15 pounds of salt a year." American Heart Association, *American Heart Association Low-Salt Cookbook* (New York: Random House, 2009). Available online: http://books.google.com/books?id=0oHTMTBKSrUC&pg=PT443&lpg=PT443&dq=5800+milligrams+of+sodium&source=bl&ots=Sthrb0RkQF&sig=tpYZfhXWLAYG-JbnYKNPzhvafr0&hl=en&sa=X&ei=S_lNUp24C6LXyAH62ICADQ&ved=0CDwQ6AEwAw#v=onepage&q=5800%20milligrams%20&f=false.

page 38, "...the calories we eat in this country." Institute of Food Technologists, research presented at the 2011 Institute of Food Technologists (IFT) Annual Meeting & Food Expo. Available online: http://www.ift.org/newsroom/news-releases/2011/june/20/snacking-constitutes-25-percent-of-calories-consumed-in-us.aspx.

page 43, "...you really only need about 225 grams a day." "Healthy Diet: Do You Follow Dietary Guidelines?," http://www.mayoclinic.org/how-to-eat-healthy/art-20046590.

page 45, "...comes from processed foods." Ryssdal, "Processed Foods Make 70 Percent of the US Diet."

page 45, "...nearly any other country in the world (except Mexico, which just passed us)? Obesity!" Food and Agriculture Organization of the United Nations, The State of Food and Agriculture, 2013. Available online: http://www.fao.org/docrep/018/i3300e/i3300e.pdf.

page 45, "...80 percent of our processed foods." Non-GMO Project, http://www.nongmoproject.org/learn-more/gmos-and-your-family/.

Chapter 3

page 51, "...actually preferred the cookies to cocaine." "Student-faculty research suggests Oreos can be compared to drugs of abuse in lab rats," Connecticut College News, October 15, 2013. Available online: http://www.conncoll.edu/news/news-archive/2013/student-faculty-research-shows-oreos-are-just-as-addictive-as-drugs-in-lab-rats-.htm#.UoqVtI1uFvP.

page 66, "...and just 4 percent on fruit." Beth Hoffman, "One Way to Be Healthier: Don't Eat like the Average American," Forbes, March 18, 2013, http://www.forbes.com/sites/bethhoffman/2013/03/18/one-way-to-be-healthier-dont-eat-like-the-average-american/.

page 72, "...who got a solid 7 hours of shut-eye a night!" S. R. Patel and F. B. Hu, "Short Sleep Duration and Weight Gain: A Systematic Review," *Obesity (Silver Spring)* 16 (2008): 643–53; S. R. Patel et al., "Association between Reduced Sleep and Weight Gain in Women," *American Journal of Epidemiology* 164 (2006): 947–54.

Part 2

Chapter 4

page 83, "...but because they no longer liked it!" Food and Health with Timi Gustafson, http://www.timigustafson.com/2012/taste-bud-rehab/.

Chapter 5

page 94, "...through conditions like type 2 diabetes and heart disease." Dariush Mozaffarian et al., research presented at the American Heart Association's Epidemiology and Prevention/Nutrition, Physical Activity and Metabolism 2013 Scientific Sessions.

page 94, "It's relevant for ALL of us, no matter our age." Healthy Child, http://www.healthychild.com/10-reasons-to-keep-kids-off-soda/.

page 95, "...85 fewer calories during the meal." E. A. Dennis et al., "Water Consumption Increases Weight Loss during a Hypocaloric Diet Intervention in Middle-age and Older Adults," Obesity 18, no. 2 (February 2010): 300–307. doi: 10.1038/oby.2009.235. Epub August 6, 2009. http://www.ncbi.nlm.nih.gov/pubmed/19661958.

page 96, ". . . stayed elevated for more than an hour." Michael Boschmann et al., "Water-induced Thermogenesis," *Journal of Clinical Endocrinology & Metabolism* 88, no. 12: 6015–19. Copyright © 2003 by The Endocrine Society.

page 105, ". . . end up with type 2 diabetes by 7 percent." R. B. Hu et al., "Television Watching and Other Sedentary Behaviors in Relation to Risk of Obesity and Type 2 Diabetes Mellitus in Women," JAMA 289, no. 14 (April 9, 2003): 1785–91.

page 105, ". . . no matter how fit you are." P. T. Katzmarzyk et al., "Sitting Time and Mortality from All Causes, Cardiovascular Disease, and Cancer," Medicine and Science in Sports and Exercise 4, no. 5 (May 2009): 998–1005. doi: 10.1249/MSS.0b013e3181930355.

Chapter 8

page 132, ". . . when we eat chocolate cake!" J. Moll et al., "Human Fronto-Mesolimbic Networks Guide Decisions about Charitable Donation," *Proceedings of the National Academy of Sciences 103, no. 42 (October 17, 2006): 15623–28.*

page 132, ". . . when we eat chocolate cake!" D. Tankersley et al., "Altruism Is Associated with an Increased Response to Agency," *Nature Neuroscience* 10, no. 2 (February 2007): 150–51.

Part 3

Chapter 10

page 152, ". . . to make your Sugar Savvy meals and drinks." The food lists in this chapter were adapted from the American Diabetes Association Exchange Lists for Meal Planning. Food portion sizes were also developed based on data obtained from: the USDA National Nutrient Database for Standard Reference (Release 26 available on-line at: http://ndb.nal.usda.gov/ndb/search/list) and Bowe's and Church's Food Values of Portions Commonly Used,19th edition by Jean A.T. Pennington, PhD, RD and Judith Spungen, MS, RD (Wolters Kluwer Lippincott Williams and Wilkins, 2010).

page 163, ". . .46 grams per day for adult women." USDA Dietary Guidelines for Americans, 2010, http://www.health.gov/dietaryguidelines/2010.asp.

page 169, ". . . plus research shows they can help you lose weight!" Zhu et al., "Calcium Plus Vitamin D3 Supplementation Facilitated Fat Loss in Overweight and Obese College Students with Very-Low Calcium Consumption: A Randomized Controlled Trial," *Nutrition Journal* 12, no. 8 (January 8, 2013). doi: 10.1186/1475-2891-12-8. http://www.ncbi.nlm.nih.gov/pubmed/23297844.

page 187, ". . .soy beans, tofu, and more." USDA National Nutrient Database for Standard Reference, Release 25, "Calcium, Ca mg ( ) Content of Selected Foods per Common Measure, sorted by nutrient content," https://www.ars.usda.gov/SP2UserFiles/Place/12354500/Data/SR25/nutrlist/sr25w301.pdf.

Chapter 12

page 226, ". . . developing prediabetes or diabetes dropped 12 percent." P. Srikanthan and A. S. Karlamangla, "Relative Muscle Mass Is Inversely Associated with Insulin Resistance and Prediabetes. Findings from the Third National Health and Nutrition Examination Survey," *The Journal of Clinical Endocrinology & Metabolism* 96, no. 9 (September 2011): 2898–2903. doi: 10.1210/jc.2011-0435. Epub July 21, 2011. http://www.ncbi.nlm.nih.gov/pubmed/21778224.

INDEX